The Doctor

methuen | drama

LONDON • NEW YORK • OXFORD • NEW DELHI • SYDNEY

METHUEN DRAMA
Bloomsbury Publishing Plc
50 Bedford Square, London, WC1B 3DP, UK
1385 Broadway, New York, NY 10018, USA
29 Earlsfort Terrace, Dublin 2, Ireland

BLOOMSBURY, METHUEN DRAMA and the Methuen Drama logo are
trademarks of Bloomsbury Publishing Plc

First published in Great Britain 2019 by Oberon Books
This edition published by Methuen Drama 2022

Cover design: James Illman

A catalogue record for this book is available from the British Library.

A catalog record for this book is available from the Library of Congress.

ISBN: PB: 978-1-350-38254-1
      ePDF: 978-1-350-38256-5
      eBook: 978-1-350-38255-8

Series: Modern Plays

Printed and bound in Great Britain

The purpose of poetry is to remind us
how difficult it is to remain just one person,
for our house is open, there are no keys in the doors,
and invisible guests come in and out at will.
(**from *Ars Poetica?* by Czeslaw Milosz**)

Acknowledgements

My greatest debt is to the actors and creative team of the original production, whose ideas, instincts and input quite literally create the show, and to all of whom I am genuinely grateful. For many of them, their involvement precedes this script – and theirs is the first thank you and the biggest.

Another team of actors read a draft of the play and offered their thoughts and encouragement at an early stage of development – to them, much thanks, and a heartfelt thank you to the exceptional Julia Horan, whose role in creating a production before it even knows itself cannot be underestimated.

Many other people kindly spoke to me, answered my questions, shared their expertise, and offered thoughts and notes on the script in its various drafts – including Helen Lewis, Rachel Taylor, Helena Clark, Stephen Grosz, Ben Naylor, Ilinca Radulian, Branden Jacobs-Jenkins, Anne Washburn, Chris Campbell, Adam Crossley, Adam Kay, Daniel Sokol, Jonathan Freedland, Josh Higgott, Rupert Goold, Lucy Pattison, Emma Pritchard, Rebecca Frecknall, Stephanie Bain, Alexander Scott, Judith Beniston, Emily Vaughan-Barratt, Anastasia Bruce-Jones, Ingoh Brux, Duncan Macmillan and Zara Tempest-Walters. Thank you all and apologies, and thanks, to anyone I've forgotten.

RI, August 2019

Characters

This play was originally produced at the Almeida Theatre, where it had its first performance on 10th August, 2019.

Cast (in alphabetical order)
Oliver Alvin-Wilson
Nathalie Armin
Paul Higgins
Mariah Louca
Pamela Nomvete
Daniel Rabin
Joy Richardson
Kirsty Rider
Juliet Stevenson
Naomi Wirthner
Ria Zmitrowicz

Creative Team

Direction	Robert Icke
Design	Hildegard Bechtler
Light	Natasha Chivers
Sound and Composition	Tom Gibbons
Associate Costume Design	Deborah Andrews
Additional Composition	Hannah Ledwidge
Casting	Julia Horan CDG
Resident Director	TD Moyo
Costume Supervision	Megan Doyle
Photography	Manuel Harlan
Company Stage Manager	Claire Sibley
Deputy Stage Manager	Bethan McKnight
Assistant Stage Manager	Beth Cotton
Bioethics Consultant	Daniel Sokol

The production (eventually) transferred to the Duke of York's Theatre, London, where it played its first performance on 29th September, 2022.

Cast (in alphabetical order)
Christopher Osikanlu Colquhoun
Doña Croll
Juliet Garricks
Mark Hammersley
Preeya Kalidas
Takiyah Kamaria
Hannah Ledwidge
Mariah Louca
John Mackay
Celia Nelson
Daniel Rabin
Juliet Stevenson
Diana Thomas
Matilda Tucker
Naomi Wirthner
Sabrina Wu

A note on the text

A forward slash (/) marks the point of interruption of overlapping dialogue.

A comma on a separate line

,

indicates a pause, a rest, a silence, an upbeat or a lift. Length and intensity are context dependent.

Square brackets [like this] indicates words which are part of the intention of the line but which are not spoken aloud.

A * on a separate line denotes a change of scene or a time-jump. They should feel like the change of (or the loss of) a train of thought for RUTH but mostly the dialogue should continue uninterrupted.

A note on the casting

Actors' identities should be carefully considered in the casting of the play. In all sections except for *Take the Debate,* each actor's identity should be directly dissonant with their character's in at least one way. Sometimes these dissonances are specifically designated in the text, sometimes it's up to the production – but the acting should hold the mystery until the play reveals it. The idea is that the audience are made to re-consider characters (and events) as they learn more about who the characters are.

This text went to press before the production opened and so may differ slightly from what was performed. But let's not worry too much about that.

RUTH   which

which is it

Hello, yes, sorry – my name is Ruth Wolff, double-f

which is it (god, you'd think I'd know this)

which is it I need if someone's died? a body, yes –

no, not urgent – I'm sure. yes. Yes. I'm crystal clear.

I'm a doctor

*

CHARLIE speaks: THE FIRST DAY

CHARLIE is about the same age as RUTH. It's important that the audience are never told explicitly whether the character is male or female.

A room in the Elizabeth Institute. MURPHY and HARDIMAN come in to a room where JUNIOR waits.

MURPHY	We were playing as a team – I mean, we played better than we've been playing –
JUNIOR	do you know where Professor Hardiman is?
MURPHY	. . . that's him
HARDIMAN	You're the new junior
JUNIOR	Yes –
HARDIMAN	Roger Hardiman, senior consultant, deputy director – [without stopping]
JUNIOR	Oh – I'm / my name's
HARDIMAN	there's supposed to be a report, autopsy, three days ago, male mid-70s
JUNIOR	It's here, it's just come in –

JUNIOR passes it, HARDIMAN takes it and reads

HARDIMAN	It was his liver. She was right.

HARDIMAN goes, furious, leaving the report behind

MURPHY	Which means: I'm now owed money.
JUNIOR	You bet on patients?
MURPHY	Absolutely not. Patient was Hardiman's, very sick, we can't work out whether it's his liver or his kidneys and patient's too

weak for us to treat both – he calls the BB
in for an opinion – the BB has her Jedi
perception. Professor, says the BB, I have
nothing but my intuition, it is not my name
above the bed, but I am crystal clear that
the patient's kidneys are not the problem.
Hardiman disagrees, treats the kidneys,
patient dies. That's a fish, isn't it, your
tattoo –

JUNIOR   is that a title? The BB?

MURPHY   It's a person. Sort of. Professor Wolff. BB =
                  Big Bad

JUNIOR   Professor Wolff is my consultant

HARDIMAN   Good luck. Woman in name only.

JUNIOR   What does that mean?

HARDIMAN   It's a joke.

COPLEY comes in

COPLEY   Is Ruth here?

MURPHY   She's on her round, I think –

COPLEY   ok. They need her downstairs.

COPLEY goes out again

HARDIMAN   Do you go to pharmacology lectures?

JUNIOR   It's not Professor Creswell at the moment –

HARDIMAN   I know that.

JUNIOR   He's off on sick, so Doctor Feinman is
                  filling in.

HARDIMAN   I *know* that. But have you been to them?

3

JUNIOR   Yes –

HARDIMAN   And how are they?

JUNIOR   How are they?

HARDIMAN   Yes

JUNIOR   Good.

HARDIMAN looks at JUNIOR as if to say 'Say more'

                She gets a bit excited.

HARDIMAN   I quite agree

As MURPHY makes to go

MURPHY   BB will need to see that report. And Copley
                is looking for her –

JUNIOR   For who?

RUTH enters, overhearing

RUTH   For whom.

                For whom is Doctor Copley looking? In the
                case that you care about language at all.
                Either way, I believe I am the answer.

JUNIOR doesn't really know how to respond, HARDIMAN saves

HARDIMAN   Report's in. It was his liver. You were right.

RUTH   No, *we* were wrong. We are one institution,
                Roger, not a balkanised set of opinions –
                and here, we got it wrong. Could I have
                that report, please?

JUNIOR   This one?

RUTH	That one. In my hand. Thank you.
	,
	I wouldn't join the boys' club just yet. You may have better options.
JUNIOR	Actually I'm with your firm again today, Professor
RUTH	I do not run a 'firm'. Coming through the doors of this institute, we might have cleaning firms, or firms of engineers – solicitors' firms, occasionally, but I run a medical *team.*
JUNIOR	Sure
RUTH	Good. There's a patient in room one, female, fourteen years old, sepsis, antibiotics aren't achieving source control. There's a nurse in there who needs relieving. The parents are on their way here, but someone should be with her at all times. Could you take over?
MURPHY	Why have we got a dying fourteen year old / in an Alzheimer's institute
RUTH	Because I was in A+E when she was brought in and sometimes, Paul, though try not to let this astonish you, doctors treat patients. *(Seamlessly to J.)* She's maximal analgesia, GCS is 9, so she's only half-conscious. Notes are up to date. Bleep me if anything changes. Yes? Go.

JUNIOR goes. RUTH glances over the report

| HARDIMAN | You been here all night? |

RUTH	Yes, with that patient, trying to get antibiotics to work.
HARDIMAN	I can take over if you need to get some rest?
MURPHY	It's basically over
RUTH	It is over when there is a body and not a single second before. Doctor Murphy, have we cured dementia? Is there nowhere for you to be?
MURPHY	Speaking of bodies, I think we're about to be looking for a new head of pharmacology –
RUTH	Yes. I visited Professor Creswell this weekend. He isn't going to be coming back. In either sense.
MURPHY	Ah. Shame. I think we might be able to persuade Bob Munro.
RUTH	I'm sure we could. But why would we want to?

MURPHY goes. HARDIMAN refers to the report, which RUTH is reading.

HARDIMAN	I should have listened to you, Ruth, you called it absolutely / right
RUTH	One of us had to be right and you followed your instincts. Nothing to be ashamed of there. Patients do die.

COPLEY enters

COPLEY	Someone here to see your sepsis patient –
RUTH	No visitors
COPLEY	I think [he's immediate family]

6

RUTH	No visitors. Patient's only half with us.
COPLEY	He's making quite a fuss – I think he's immediate family
RUTH	He can't be, they're out of the country.
COPLEY	Okay

COPLEY goes. RUTH carries on reading the report.

,

HARDIMAN	I really do apologise, Ruth, about / the
RUTH	I'm not reading this to humiliate you, Roger. I'm reading it because I need to have read it.
JUNIOR	Professor –
RUTH *(chorus)*	Yes?
HARDIMAN *(chorus)*	Yes?
JUNIOR	Wolff, sorry – Professor – she's saying her boyfriend's coming – the patient is / saying
RUTH	He isn't. He isn't here, he never was. She's been saying that all night.
HARDIMAN	If you want me to take over, Ruth, see her through to the end –
JUNIOR	She's – going to die?
RUTH	It's not over 'til there's a body. You know what – I'm going to come back down.

*

RUTH and JUNIOR have happened upon COPLEY and the FATHER. The FATHER is played by a white actor.

RUTH	Why are we all standing outside my patient's door?
COPLEY	I'm sorry, Professor – I didn't want to call security but this gentleman is insistent he sees your patient –
RUTH	You are not wearing a lanyard. A *badge*, I mean
FATHER	no – (?)
RUTH	I take your point, it's a flawed system, it's a naïve sort of logic, really, that says a rogue gunman might be made conspicuous because he's the only person in the hospital *not* to be wearing ID – could I take your name, Mr –
FATHER	Father –

A beat

RUTH	Forgive me: I was told Emily's parents were on a plane and / wouldn't be here for a couple / of hours [at least]
FATHER	No it's Father – Father Jacob. I'm a priest.
RUTH	I'm afraid Emily isn't up to visitors.
COPLEY	I've told him that, Professor –
FATHER	They said she is conscious
RUTH	She is –
FATHER	Which is surely a good sign
COPLEY	I think we're beyond signs.

8

RUTH	Thank you, Michael – could you check on the patient, please?
FATHER	She is going to die?
RUTH	As are we all.

RUTH makes to move on. The FATHER puts on a dog collar.

FATHER	Her parents asked me – Emily's parents – suggested she might need me to be here. They phoned me from the airport.
RUTH	Well, they didn't phone me.
FATHER	With respect, Doctor, that's not my problem.
	,
RUTH	Emily's blood pressure is extremely low. That means a real chance of a cardiac event which means we can't risk interventions. Our focus of care at this moment is comfort.
FATHER	Mine too
RUTH	I'm sorry, I don't understand
FATHER	Let me make it clearer. Emily is gravely ill. Emily's parents asked me to be here and to attend to her. Is that not obvious?
RUTH	It's obvious when the patient has requested religious assistance, because it's written on her medical notes. In this instance, there's nothing of the sort.
FATHER	So –
RUTH	So no visitors.

FATHER	I'm not a visitor
RUTH	Then who are you?
FATHER	Doctor, Emily's parents are Catholic, her parents are members of my congregation and they / asked me to be here –
COPLEY	Ruth, do you want me to call / the parents?
RUTH	They're on a plane. And it isn't their decision. So Emily is religious?
FATHER	Yes

He's not 100% certain, somehow

RUTH	And she attends your church?
FATHER	Her parents do.
RUTH	Not her?
FATHER	She has done, yes

,

RUTH	I'm sorry, sir, but I have / no
FATHER	[sir] Father
RUTH	I have no way of knowing whether she last attended church in a Christening gown. The only thing of relevance is what she herself believes – and I don't know. I don't know if you've ever met her.

The FATHER's eyes are blazing but he doesn't raise his voice.

FATHER	I'm a liar, then

,

	Shall we go in and ask Emily?
RUTH	No. She isn't expecting your visit, she hasn't asked for your visit, and she's delirious. She's dreaming. She only half knows she's here, in a hospital – but she thinks she's going to be fine. And I am crystal clear that if we snap her out of that state, we cause significant distress. You let her know she's dying, then she panics, that means physiological stress, more demand on her circulation and a number of other things she simply isn't able to cope with.
FATHER	What are you saying?
RUTH	I'm saying you walk in there like the grim reaper and there is no way that she, in her current condition, can die without panic and / distress
FATHER	I wonder what it is about me that you think I'm so incompetent / that

MURPHY arrives to the scene

MURPHY	Professor, can / I borrow you –
RUTH	One minute, Paul –
FATHER	I'm sorry: is there any chance she might be cured?
COPLEY	No.
RUTH	There's always a chance
FATHER	Do you know the cause of her condition?
RUTH	Yes, I do

FATHER	And?
RUTH	*And* I'd need her consent to reveal it to you. And I'd rather not have this conversation out here in front of an audience – Doctor Copley, could you find an empty / room
FATHER	So she could die within the hour. She can't be cured. But you're telling me she can't receive the last rites?
RUTH	It's my name above her bed. And it is my duty to protect my patient –
FATHER	From what?
RUTH	and act in her best interests
FATHER	Protect her from what?
RUTH	From an unpeaceful death
	,
FATHER	But she has the right to make her own choice
RUTH	I'm going to leave this now, and go back in

Quietly, JUNIOR leaves to the patient – this starts to really escalate. CYPRIAN comes in.

FATHER	I thought you couldn't help her –
RUTH	We don't only attend the patients we can help – and I don't have to justify myself to you
FATHER	If she can see you, she can see me –
RUTH	Not here. Not how it works.
CYPRIAN	Professor, is everything all right here?

RUTH	It's fine
FATHER	Sorry, are you her supervisor?
CYPRIAN	what?
FATHER	I want to speak to her supervisor
RUTH	I hate to burst your bubble but I'm the Founding Director of this Institute, so my supervisor is either the board or the General Medical Council and you don't have that kind of time –
COPLEY	Professor, I think we need to calm / down
RUTH	I'm calm. We're finished here.
FATHER	I'm not finished here. What happens if I walk calmly through that door?
RUTH	Then my colleagues here will call security –
CYPRIAN	We would have to / call security
FATHER	Listen, mate, keep out of this. Are you forbidding me / from entering this room?
RUTH	What are you doing?

The FATHER has started a recording device, he speaks into it

FATHER	I'm recording what's left of our conversation
RUTH	In which case I'm going to terminate it.
FATHER	I'm now going to walk calmly into Emily's room, Doctor – I'm sorry, can you get out of my way –
RUTH	You have *zero* authority here. I don't know who the hell you are. You want to get uppity

	with me, then fine. But you're wasting your time because there is really no way I'm going to let you near that child
MURPHY	Professor, I think / we should
FATHER	I'm now going to walk into the room –
RUTH	There is a child in there, father, about to die a peaceful death and she needs my full attention as a matter of urgency to keep that death peaceful –

As the FATHER moves to the door, RUTH touches him. The FATHER throws her hand off. Probably this shouldn't be naturalistically dramatized: that is, we shouldn't be shown exactly what happens.

FATHER	Get your hands off me – don't you dare TOUCH me, don't you DARE.
JUNIOR	*(From within.)* Doctor Wolff – hello? Can you come in here, please? Quick

The kettle starts to boil. A repeating ding-dong alarm noise perhaps sounds too, as if a machine is reporting a patient in distress. JUNIOR re-enters.

	Doctor – she's panicking – heart-rate's skyrocketing
RUTH	Why?
JUNIOR	She says she doesn't want to die
FATHER	I thought she didn't know – (!)
RUTH	She didn't know. She didn't.
*	
CHARLIE	You touched him. The priest

RUTH	Yes –
CHARLIE	How did you touch him?
RUTH	I put my hand on his shoulder
CHARLIE	Was it a touch or a shove? Or a push? Did it have force?
RUTH	I –
	no. It was a touch. I mean, as if the word itself is material to / the
CHARLIE	If I were your lawyer and not your partner, these are the questions I'd ask you in the first ten minutes –
RUTH	I hate the word partner. It sounds like we're – accountants.

*

The doctors re-enter the corridor where the FATHER waits.

FATHER	Can I go in there now? I need to see Emily / before
JUNIOR	I'm afraid it's too late –
RUTH	*Time*, please
JUNIOR	Time of death eleven minutes past eight.
RUTH	Thank you – everyone

The doctors are aware of the FATHER, not moving – perhaps emotional

COPLEY	[is] cause of death – sepsis arising from complications of termination of pregnancy?
RUTH	[just put] Sepsis.

The FATHER turns around. He looks at RUTH.

MURPHY   I'm sorry things got so heated before, Father –

FATHER   You idiots

                you don't get to grant absolution. What's
                happened here is is is a very serious thing

COPLEY   Ok – ok –

FATHER   I trust you won't have a problem if I attend
                to Emily now, Ms Wolff.

RUTH   Professor Wolff

The FATHER storms out.

MURPHY   You're out of line. You should have let him
                in.

RUTH   To remind you of the basic rule, you get to
                call the shots, Doctor Murphy, when the
                nurse writes your name above the patient's
                bed. Are you having trouble with your
                reading?

MURPHY   We'll see. We'll see.

MURPHY exits

*

The kettle clicks off, boiled. We're in RUTH's house.

CHARLIE   And you watched the girl die

RUTH   Yes. Screaming for her parents and
                scratching the nurse and I don't want to
                die I don't want to die – five minutes before
                she's floating hazy in a dream and she dies
                trying to tear through a nightmare

CHARLIE	Not the first one you've lost, Ruthie
RUTH	No
CHARLIE	Tea?
RUTH	No thank you
	She was fourteen.
	Is someone in the house?
CHARLIE	Your friend's upstairs.
RUTH	Oh?
CHARLIE	You gave her keys, remember. What did the girl die of?
RUTH	Self-administered abortion. She'd hoped she wasn't pregnant for four months. Parents went away for the week, she'd got the pills online, took them probably two days ago, it's an incomplete abortion, bleeding, she ignores it, tries to stem the bleed with pads, didn't work, falls unconscious, hours pass, her friend's mum finds her, gets her into us, but by that point she's already far gone with sepsis.
	And none of this story is clear until after she's dead.
(Deep: if only.)	If they'd let her have a civilised abortion in a medical setting, she'd be eating ice-cream and surfing the internet.
CHARLIE	who's they?
RUTH	Catholic parents.
*	

SAMI	Your cat is quite weird. It has like a proper attitude problem. Last ten times I've been here it's nowhere to be seen and then today it's like sitting on the landing and it's like staring at me, like 'hi'. It looks at you like it knows your secrets.
RUTH	perhaps it does
SAMI	is it a he-cat or a she-cat?
RUTH	it's a cat-cat
SAMI	But it's got a name – (?)
RUTH	Astonishingly, in nine years it's never introduced itself in English –
SAMI	It doesn't have a name – (!)
RUTH	Oh it'll happily ignore a whole variety of names.
SAMI	I am like – appalled –
RUTH	Having spent all day with an abortion patient, I'm *like* philosophical about the things people choose to humanise
SAMI	I thought it was all like Alzheimer's at your institute –
RUTH	It is. But I saw the girl come in and sometimes, something else takes over and I was taking her up to the Institute before I'd even – you know what, this doesn't matter.
SAMI	Your kettle is always boiled.
RUTH	It reminds me I'm alive. You want tea?
SAMI	I don't do tea. Or coffee.

RUTH	You don't *do* them?
SAMI	You are literally doing my head in, language police.

Perhaps CHARLIE makes RUTH a cup of tea

RUTH	Tea was the currency of love in our house, growing up. The transmission of affection in a chipped mug. And a biscuit, if you were really in favour.
SAMI	How long have you lived here?
RUTH	For ever.
	,
SAMI	When I was a kid, people used to call this house the witch's cottage.

SAMI senses potential hurt in RUTH and saves it

	Because it's near the wood. And it's old.
RUTH	And there's a black cat.
	,
	Is that school work you're doing?
SAMI	*(Sarc)* No, I look at circle theorems to, like, relax
RUTH	To *like* relax
SAMI	What would you say?
RUTH	It's the 'likes', everything is – comparative. Nothing contained. No thought *finished.*
SAMI	Don't you like that? Don't you *like* that?

19

RUTH   Open-ended isn't great in medicine.
              Usually means someone's about to enter
              the past tense.

              ,

              I don't look like a witch

SAMI   You look sad.

RUTH   I suppose, in one way, I am *like* a witch.
              The process of looking at someone, at
              something about them. Extrapolating
              evidence. Guessing what will happen to
              them next. That's fortune telling. Or as we
              have it, diagnostic medicine.

SAMI   You're not a witch

RUTH   We still give you poison for cancer and
              chalk for your stomach and the bark
              of a willow tree for headaches. Only we
              write different things on the bottles. In a
              hundred years – two hundred years, they'll
              look back at us and they'll know the cure.
              It'll seem so obvious, they'll think we were
              so stupid not to know. Doctors – are witches
              in white.

              'Take this potion, my pretty one, uncork
              the bottle and drink, once at dawn, once
              at dusk and your back will straighten, your
              eyes will brighten and your dreams – will set
              themselves upright for years to come.'

SAMI   OK, witch-doctor, what if I don't?

RUTH   Then you die

SAMI	We're all going to die, though. Like – a sell-by-date for your soul. It's a 'when' not an 'if'. Could be tomorrow. Or tonight. In here.
	now
	now
RUTH	It's over when there's a body. I should find us some food. Your mum knows you're here
SAMI	If she didn't, she wouldn't care –
	Are you okay?
RUTH	oh I don't know. A girl died today. At work.

CHARLIE speaks: THE SECOND DAY

ROBERTS   The important thing is that we don't panic

CYPRIAN   She called me and she wanted to know
                 what we were doing about the situation and
                 I said, what situation, and then she tells me
                 what situation and I said well, there wasn't
                 much we could do about the situation, the
                 situation had happened and she said well
                 people really aren't very happy about it and
                 she slams the phone down

COPLEY   So what?

CYPRIAN   So she has a lot of money and she has a
                 husband who is on our board, and she also,
                 as things currently stand, has promised
                 quite a lot of her money to our new
                 building

COPLEY   She's the one who thought we should have
                 a ball. Big red woman. Met her touring the
                 research centre last year. I mean, a hospital
                 ball.

ROBERTS   Right –

            RUTH enters

COPLEY   She says 'does the hospital ever host events
                 for its donors? I think donors means
                 organ donors, and then she says 'We could
                 organize a ball' and I thought – well, good
                 luck finding a bloke to donate that –

CYPRIAN   Shall we not air our grievances to a junior
                 doctor? That woman is a development asset –

MURPHY   I spoke to development – and development
              think it's a problem.

CYPRIAN   Ruth, I've got a donor who's very unhappy
              about our priest situation –

RUTH   and I've got three questions: One, why are
              we spending time on this? Two, when did
              we start to use the word 'development' to
              mean 'us asking people for money'? Three,
              Doctor Murphy, why are you involved?

CYPRIAN   This is important, Ruth, she's unhappy. So
              what are we going to do?

RUTH   Cure unhappiness. And Rebecca is here –
              because – (?)

MURPHY   Because Rebecca is responsible for public
              relations.

RUTH   And her advice is?

ROBERTS   We shouldn't make a public response –

RUTH   Good. Let's move on.

ROBERTS   – but how does your donor know?

A pause. They look at each other.

MURPHY   I would assume it's either the parents or
              the priest. Roger Hardiman spoke to the
              parents when they arrived late last night
              and they were obviously / very upset

CYPRIAN   They'll sue

JUNIOR   For wrongful death?

ROBERTS *(chorus)*   Probably
CYPRIAN *(chorus)*   Yes – who are you?

JUNIOR	I'm / [goes to say his name but]
COPLEY	They'll lose on wrongful death. Death was inevitable.
MURPHY	Was it, though?
ROBERTS	Medically, did Ruth do anything wrong? What are the actual rules?
COPLEY	If the patient's a child, then it's up to the doctor. There was nothing on the notes about religion. No parents available to contact. No time to consult more widely. There's really nothing else Ruth could have done.
ROBERTS	[but] could she have let the priest give the girl the last rites?
MURPHY	Exactly
COPLEY	He was a man coming in off the street –
MURPHY	wearing a dog collar
COPLEY	which would be impossible to fake, you're quite right
MURPHY	He was a man of God and she basically called him a liar, I mean, why are we pretending we weren't convinced he was a priest?
RUTH	I really don't think any of us are
ROBERTS	What does the Hippocratic oath say?

'

I'm asking because other people will.

MURPHY	Brian?
CYPRIAN	No-one swears the Hippocratic oath. Not any more. It's ancient and it's therefore in the bin. The guidelines are still to 'do no harm' – but the thing that really counts is patient choice.
MURPHY	The patient wasn't told she had a choice
RUTH	The patient wasn't conscious
MURPHY	That's not what it says in the notes
RUTH	And why are you reading the notes?
CYPRIAN	OK – we need a report that confirms whether the girl would have died anyway.
RUTH	I asked for it last night. It'll be here this morning. It'll say: yes, she would have [died anyway]. Now let's move onto something important. We need to make a decision about departmental structure / in the new building –
MURPHY	Sorry, Ruth – if the parents are already going to complain, they'll say that if the girl's prognosis was hopeless, the priest should have been allowed in.
ROBERTS	And will the priest have the backing of the church?
COPLEY	Does the pope shit in the woods?
CYPRIAN	Michael, tone, please
COPLEY	Brian, I am merely pointing out that they have a habit of protecting their own

MURPHY	Like doctors, then
JUNIOR	There's a petition online
	,
RUTH	What?
MURPHY	About this? Are you on it now?
CYPRIAN	Read it. Read out what it says
JUNIOR	'The incident that took place at the Elizabeth Institute on – et cetera et cetera, Father Jacob Rice was summoned to the death-bed of Emily Ronan by her parents to give her the last rites. The consultant in charge, who is not a Christian, refused to admit the Father to the girl's bedside, on the grounds that his ministry might be damaging to the dying girl's health.'
COPLEY	But that / isn't
CYPRIAN	Let him read
JUNIOR	'The girl was dying as a result of complications after the termination of her pregnancy. The Elizabeth Institute is a private part of the hospital largely funded by a club of anonymous donors. When the Father tried to enter Emily's room, the consultant in charge used physical force and shoved him out of / the way'
COPLEY	What?
RUTH	That didn't happen –
MURPHY	Well [that definitely did happen]

CYPRIAN	There are witnesses
RUTH	There are not witnesses that / saw me
CYPRIAN	I'm saying there are witnesses, so that's not going to be a *problem*
MURPHY	Brian [I saw her push him]

CYPRIAN crushes the opposition with firm entitlement

CYPRIAN	*That is not going to be a problem.* Continue. Read.
JUNIOR	'During this fight, Emily died without receiving the last rites. We, the undersigned, are horrified at this doctor's treatment of a religious man and call for action to be taken in investigating this incident and to urgently raise the issue that Christian patients need Christian doctors.'
MURPHY	This is a mess.
RUTH	Even at the level of grammar, if that petition's anything to go by –
ROBERTS	We shouldn't respond. It's obviously political, and I don't think people will listen –
COPLEY	Spotting a spotlight and trying to leap into it – though the anti-semitic undertones…
CYPRIAN	What?
COPLEY	'A club of shady anonymous donors'
MURPHY	I disagree
COPLEY	And soon someone's going to be saying 'This is a Christian country'

MURPHY	This is a Christian country
COPLEY	Ignore it and it'll die down.
MURPHY	I disagree – our funding rests on our reputation and our reputation is about to get punched –
CYPRIAN	The timing is unfortunate, given the new building
MURPHY	so then we need to make a statement
ROBERTS	I really don't think / that's
COPLEY	It's the Catholic Church! They're not a moral arbiter!

HARDIMAN enters

HARDIMAN	Ruth, can I borrow you for a minute?
RUTH	How many signatures does it have? That petition
	,
JUNIOR	twenty-seven.
CYPRIAN	Twenty-seven? Then what the hell are you doing bringing it up? Why the hell should anyone care?
JUNIOR	I thought / it might be
RUTH	Now can we please talk about something important
CYPRIAN	This is important
RUTH	Sixty-one year old man, you really are in the danger window for a heart attack, so it really would be best if you kept calm. And

	stayed hydrated. Could we please get some water for Brian?
CYPRIAN	Look. No-one knows it's Ruth. There's no way they find out. We deal with the parents internally and we put out a neutral statement that says hospital procedures were followed
ROBERTS *(chorus)*	No –
RUTH *(chorus)*	No
MURPHY	Were they followed?
RUTH	Yes.
HARDIMAN	But if the parents / disagree
RUTH	Patient was a child, so it's for the doctor, not the parents / to decide
COPLEY	Exactly
HARDIMAN	A neutral statement isn't going to cut it. This is already bigger than that. The press love a medical ethics story, we're a wealthy institution, fair-game for punching up – science versus faith. They love all the stuff about the Jehovah's Witnesses who won't accept transfused blood
COPLEY	Exactly, people who'd rather die than accept technological progress– people frightened of a new idea, to which I say, 'Fine, you die if you want to but my kids are having vaccinations'
CYPRIAN	Can we please try and speak in a professional / manner
COPLEY	I'm saying this is not serious

CYPRIAN	This is serious
RUTH	This is the healing power of religious faith squaring up against proven, empirical, scientific medicine. The sound you're hearing is the sound you hear when an old tradition dies. When an elderly man picks a fight to prove that he still can, we smile, we walk away, we don't respond.
HARDIMAN	A tradition dying. You're really comfortable talking about religion like that?
RUTH	I really am, yes. I am not asking anyone to do anything differently. I'm not asking to be involved with their lives or for them to live according to my rules. I am asking them to let us get on with our work. So can we please get on with our work?
HARDIMAN	Religion is people's lives – for these people, their whole identity –
RUTH	Exactly. And progress beats identity every single time. Now can we please move on?
HARDIMAN	I'm a Catholic. Do you want to say that again – and to me?
RUTH	I will happily say that to you, Roger, at the point when you try to stop me having access to a patient, over whom you have no authority, and who I am trying to treat. Until then, I shall live and let live. Let's move on.
CYPRIAN	Yes, but if the press pick this up –
RUTH	Then we will cross that bridge, and if I have to, I will say my piece –

ROBERTS	I don't think we need to worry about press at this point –
RUTH	And you're [ROBERTS] in charge of press and that's good enough for me – so lets / move on
MURPHY	But not for me – I'm sorry, Ruth / but we cannot take this lightly
COPLEY	Oh take the fucking advice –
CYPRIAN	MICHAEL
HARDIMAN	Okay, we need to calm / this down
CYPRIAN *(uncalm)*	I am the CLINICAL DIRECTOR of this INSTITUTE and I have spent three bloody miserable years working us to the point of exhausting to raise the funding for this new building and I don't think it's funny that we might be jeopardised [over so little] – we have a meeting, well she has a meeting this week with the Health Secretary –
RUTH	Today, in / fact –
CYPRIAN	TODAY. So of all the hills in all the world, why choose to die on this one? We break ground on our own bespoke building in six months' time which gives us the best tools to have the best chance of being the people who cure dementia. And that could mean a Nobel Prize for her.
RUTH	*(Fast in.)* for all of us, because we are a team. Were you coming to a point, Professor Cyprian?
CYPRIAN	We cannot allow this to become a thing.

HARDIMAN	Too late. It's the morning after and there's already the board, the petition and the pro-life group –
ROBERTS	What?
RUTH	What's happened on the board?
HARDIMAN	Murmurs
ROBERTS	And the pro-life group?
HARDIMAN	E-mails from the anti-abortion people demanding a statement. It's fine, for now. But why not get ahead? Prepare a statement – perhaps only internally, that can be circulated to the board, offered perhaps to the parents, if needs be.
RUTH	A statement saying what?
CYPRIAN	'I'm sorry if any offence was caused'
ROBERTS	You can't say 'sorry if'
MURPHY	'Sorry if' is no different to 'go and fuck yourself'
ROBERTS	Also you can't be sorry for them being offended, you have to be sorry for what you did
RUTH	I think the lack of my having done something makes that really quite difficult
HARDIMAN	'I got it wrong. I'm sorry.'
	,
	I was being her
RUTH	I didn't get it wrong

MURPHY	Wait. You think this autopsy report will say the girl would have died regardless.
RUTH	Yes. I'm crystal clear.
MURPHY	Then she *could* have had the last rites and nothing would have changed.
RUTH	Except a deeply distressing final few minutes alive –
HARDIMAN	which *is* what actually happened.
COPLEY	Can the autopsy tell us whether she was a Christian?
JUNIOR	I don't think that's funny
COPLEY	And I don't think I'm going to take censure from a junior fucking doctor. Can you go and do your rounds please?
HARDIMAN	Ruth, could I – sorr/y

The JUNIOR goes

ROBERTS	Was she a Christian?

MURPHY *(chorus)*	Yes
COPLEY *(chorus)*	No
HARDIMAN *(chorus)*	Well –

MURPHY	She was wearing a crucifix
COPLEY	That's a generational thing, loads of young / people
MURPHY	when she died, she was wearing / a crucifix
RUTH	Exactly. We don't know. We will now never know. Her parents were Catholics
HARDIMAN	are Catholics

33

COPLEY   But the point is a single case cannot be
                    blown up into a symbolic campaign /
                    against religion

HARDIMAN   Yes it can. Yes it can.

CYPRIAN suddenly has an idea

CYPRIAN   Hang on but you're religious [Ruth]

RUTH   I'm not

CYPRIAN   I thought you were Jewish

COPLEY   Not religiously Jewish

RUTH   that's right, not Jewish. My parents were
                    Jewish. They were religious people: I am
                    not.

CYPRIAN   right.

                    ,

MURPHY   But you would have been thought of as
                    Jewish – in the 1940s.

COPLEY   *(!)* Jesus Christ

MURPHY   What? That's the truth, isn't it?

RUTH   It is Paul, yes, but I think Michael's point is
                    that maybe there might be more sensitive
                    ways to reflect on the Jewish identity than
                    the ones pioneered by the Nazis. *(COPLEY is
                    ready to interrupt.)* Thank you, Michael, yes,
                    you and I lost grandparents in that war, and
                    they had stars sewn onto their lapels, but
                    their legacy is this: we now get to choose
                    what defines us – so can we please get on
                    with our lives.

CYPRIAN has been thinking about the statement

CYPRIAN	How about 'The Elizabeth Institute takes seriously any complaint, and in this instance we find / no cause'
ROBERTS	Not 'we'
COPLEY	What's wrong with we?
ROBERTS	Every 'we' implies a 'they'. It's like tacitly – you lot are making a huge fuss about nothing and we in here think it's hilarious –
HARDIMAN	Ruth, could I [borrow you]?

*

HARDIMAN	Sorry to pull you out of there, Ruth –
RUTH	It's not a problem
HARDIMAN	Good. I'm a bit worried that people could interpret this as you trying to make your point. With the priest.
RUTH	My point?
HARDIMAN	Putting faith in its place, below medicine. Religion is ancient, medicine is modern.
RUTH	Candles versus electricity, you mean?
HARDIMAN	I think candles might still exist, Ruth
RUTH	Not lighting many homes, though, are they, now: more sort of decorative knick-knacks
HARDIMAN	You know as well as I do, it's not ideal timing for a controversy.
RUTH	I do know that, yes

HARDIMAN	And the board are / wobbling –
RUTH	We'll have to see how it plays out
HARDIMAN	We could do that. But it is the whole institute that's involved, here, Ruth, not only you –
RUTH	I am aware of that, Roger
HARDIMAN	So the best thing would be to calm things down before they begin –
RUTH	Which is almost by definition difficult to do
HARDIMAN	But not here. All we need is for people to know that you had no intention of beginning some sort of anti-religious crusade –
RUTH	And you really think people have to be told that?
HARDIMAN	No. Shown.

,

	The executive meets this week. And now, given Creswell's health, we're going to have to appoint a new head of pharmacology.
RUTH	Ah
HARDIMAN	And there are two serious contenders.
RUTH	One of whom is an excellent doctor

,

HARDIMAN	I didn't know pharmacology was your specialism, Professor –

RUTH	I know you love playing charades, Roger, but I've read the materials, same as you – so can we be direct? Doctor Feinman's articles are exceptional where Doctor Munro simply lists case histories one after the other until this reader grinds her teeth. Doctor Feinman is a current employee, she knows us, knows the department: the advantage of institutional knowledge.
HARDIMAN	Some people think his case histories are excellent – and that her articles, though bursting with ideas, are over-excited and well – under-controlled. And personality-wise, for a head of department, a steadier hand / might
RUTH	It's not up to us, though, is it – the appointment is voted for by the exec
HARDIMAN	Which will split fifty-fifty, I think
RUTH	We'll see
HARDIMAN	And if it does, it's your deciding vote.
RUTH	I really am fully conversant with the procedures of this institute, Professor
HARDIMAN	Let's not get emotional, Ruth. Creswell said he would endorse Munro as his successor, said it'd be good to have a black man in that job.
RUTH	Well yes, he's a man, he doesn't want her to be promoted and prove a better HOD than him – which is exactly what will happen.
HARDIMAN	'He's a man'. It's a bit tedious, Ruth, after a while

RUTH	And so is Creswell's carping especially when one considers that the majority of what he's published in the last five years has been largely Janet Feinman's work.
HARDIMAN	And you'll say that to his face, will you?
RUTH	I don't have an issue with honesty. Shall we be straight with each other, Professor? Whether or not it's to calm the flames, you want to appoint Munro because he's a Christian.
	,
HARDIMAN	And it looks *good* to hire a *black man* in that job. I think it's our best move, Ruth.
RUTH	Right.
HARDIMAN	I could just as well say you want to appoint Feinman because she's *not* a Christian.
RUTH	But I appointed you. And Creswell. Both subscribers to the Christian religion.
HARDIMAN	'Believers', Ruth, it's not a magazine. And we are the exception, in this Institute, Professor, not the rule.
RUTH	There's not a rule
HARDIMAN	We're seen as a closed shop, Ruth.
RUTH	However we're seen, that's not what we are.
HARDIMAN	Thought experiment. We announce we're appointing Munro, we make it clear that he is a Christian and in our current crisis, subtly but definitely things calm / down

RUTH	The appointment is subject to a vote of the executive committee
HARDIMAN	I'm not asking you to vote for a fool. I think he's the better doctor.
RUTH	And I'm sure he'll be devastated it's not your deciding vote –
HARDIMAN	OK, Ruth. This is becoming a serious thing. I am being asked questions. From significant people. About this incident. And I'm very confident that those people will take the news of Munro's appointment as a clear suggestion that there's nothing here to find.
	,
	Think about it. We'll talk it through again before tomorrow –
RUTH	No need
HARDIMAN	Don't let pride get in the way, Ruth, please. And it goes without saying, all this is between us.
RUTH	No need. Tell whomever you like. Start with your noteworthy whoevers – and tell them this from me: I don't make deals.

ROBERTS enters

No wedding ring. Strange you're not married, isn't it? You live with her, don't you, but you're not married – not very Catholic.

ROBERTS	Sorry – the petition's at a touch under a hundred signatures now. Brian asked me to / tell you
RUTH	Thank you, I'm coming back, need to get on with the day. We're finished in here. Roger? Thought experiment: if I were a man, do you think you'd be dealing with this differently?
HARDIMAN	In what way differently?
RUTH	If it were a male doctor who'd handled the priest as I did.
HARDIMAN	You're suggesting that, as a man, my Y chromosome might be causing early-onset blindness and making me unconsciously deal with this crisis through a fog of misogyny? No, Ruth, I don't think I am. We are all entitled to our opinion. Aren't we? All of us. I'll keep in touch today.

HARDIMAN goes

ROBERTS	Can I speak freely?
RUTH	Go on
ROBERTS	He's an anti-Semitic prick.
RUTH	oh that's simplistic –
ROBERTS	I mean it –
RUTH	I know – but there's really a huge plurality of ways in which Roger Hardiman is a patronising moron, so I'm saying let's not just focus on the anti-Semitism with so many other irons in the fire. You're Jewish, aren't you?

ROBERTS	Yes indeed. Can I speak freely again?
RUTH	You can.
ROBERTS	Why is he still working here?
RUTH	Because he is a good doctor and if someone had to cut into my brain, I'd want him.
ROBERTS	Even though / he
RUTH	Yep. If someone has to cut open my brain, I want the best. and he is a deplorable human being, but he is also the best. There you have it. Life's complicated.
REBECCA	Are you holding up?
RUTH	It takes years to build an institution from nothing. We have nearly five hundred members of staff. To most of them, it's always been here. It's a fixture. I can only ever think of it as vulnerable.

*

CHARLIE	Not like you to be home
RUTH	Home for lunch
CHARLIE	And yet – no food
RUTH	I needed space.

,

CHARLIE	It might be the moment to bring me up.
RUTH	At work? They don't get my life. They don't get to be involved.
CHARLIE	– they don't get to know about me.

41

RUTH	what?
CHARLIE	you know
RUTH	and why would I not talk about you?
CHARLIE	because you are ashamed of the way it makes you seem.
RUTH	I'm afraid I have to dissent –
CHARLIE	I do not have a place in the story you tell the world about Ruth Wolff, and nor have I ever had one.
RUTH	I'm proud of you.
CHARLIE	I know that:

CHARLIE *(chorus)* they don't.
RUTH *(chorus)* they don't.

RUTH I go in tomorrow and start talking about you, now, it's going to seem like – like I'm asking for my 'I'm a human too' badge – some get me off the hook scheme. No. Not doing it.

CHARLIE looks at her

*

Hello?

RUTH on the phone

ROBERTS I'm sorry to phone again but they're trying to draw you out – well, someone's put out a challenge for you to step forward and defend yourself in a debate. 'The dead girl can't speak but the doctor responsible / can'

42

RUTH	I don't need to hear it –
ROBERTS	Okay. And this politics programme – you won't have watched it – debate on a hot topic, panellists interrogating the guest, they want us to send someone on. And social media is starting to heat up
RUTH	I don't need to hear what's on social media.
ROBERTS	No
	We still think the best route is silence, Ruth. This is going to blow over.

*

CYPRIAN and FLINT meet RUTH

CYPRIAN	You were a great girl then and you're a great girl now. And I'm very hopeful, we're all very hopeful, you're going to come out and fight for this old place when we need you. Funding – I mean, in terms of funding. Aren't we, Ruth? Hopeful?
RUTH	We are, Brian.
CYPRIAN	Always a pleasure to see you, my darling. I'll leave you ladies to it.

CYPRIAN goes. They look at each other.

RUTH	Minister
FLINT	Professor. It has been a while.
RUTH	I was there for your BMA speech — which I admired.

| FLINT | Then it's been a while for me. And anyway, the woman who gives the speeches is an entirely different person from the one you taught – |
| RUTH | well, they're both the most senior woman in the country now |

FLINT smiles

FLINT	It's not the job, it's what you do with it. And God there's such a lot to do. Leaky roofs and nursing numbers, sure – but then, there's monuments to build. Not merely curing patients but curing the diseases.
RUTH	I liked that line the first time too. When the woman who gives the speeches said it.
FLINT	I mean it. And I'm going to do it.
RUTH	You were always determined.
FLINT	It sounds double-edged, when you say it like that –
RUTH	I look back now and I remember things. There was one patient, you were a junior, I was a registrar perhaps, observing your consultant, anyway you're standing there with the suction pump – and you whisper to me, the treatment's wrong. We're treating the wrong thing. Anyone got anything to add?, the consultant says, he's heard your voice, he's looking straight at you. You knew. You'd told me the answer. And I looked at you – and you said nothing. And an hour later, the patient dies on the table. Because – you were right.

FLINT	That's fifteen (?) years ago –
RUTH	That's a life saved. Or not, in that instance.
FLINT	I didn't want the doctor in charge to be upstaged – I didn't want to embarrass him. Not in front of you. And it was that consultant
RUTH *(chorus)*	Henley, wasn't it?
FLINT *(chorus)*	Henley, exactly – who would write me the recommendation that would lead to my being the first woman in that hospital to get a chair, first professorship – before even your eminent self – so it could be / that...
RUTH	You think that one decision might have damaged your relationship with Henley –
FLINT	You never know. People are petty.
RUTH	You didn't put that in the manifesto
FLINT	Oh really? It was on every single page. Right there between the lines.

,

	Ruth. I understand I disappointed you. By changing course. People would rather their kids became perverts than professional politicians. I get it. But when I walk through the door of my office, there are things I can get done for medicine, more than – researching proteins or curing patients.
RUTH	We get things done here too, Jemima –
FLINT	And you're an incredible success story. Exceptional results. Though there is a

45

	sense that the Elizabeth isn't on board with the wider, how to put this, dynamics of the field. Not joining in. Elite class. Very you. And yet, year after year, you do the best research and produce the best results. And you're a woman. So there's a little envy operating. Among other things, a desire to bring you down to earth. Not that that's what this is, but that's the weather system we're standing under.
RUTH	I'm sorry, did Brian tell you about [the incident] – ?
FLINT *(obvious)*	My office briefed me this morning
RUTH *(what?)*	How did they know?
FLINT	Roger Hardiman's an ambitious little man.
RUTH	And a very good surgeon – but surely he's not [ringing round]
FLINT	his brother's now the PM's chief of staff. Came in same time I did. Phone calls are being made. And then there's the petition and so on, but for my money your real enemies live in your own house. I assume the apology's coming –
RUTH	No. It's a storm in a teacup.
FLINT	Then why take it so seriously? Pick up the teacup [and] put it in the bin. You can just close the gap between their story and yours: surf with the tide: apologise, move on. Show your staff you know how to listen –
RUTH	It's not leadership, really, though, that, is it, so much as followership

46

FLINT   What do you call a leader with no followers?

RUTH   If she's a real leader, she won't care what
             you call her.

FLINT   I like that. Might borrow it. People don't
             like you, Professor, but god do they admire
             you – a woman of integrity. I say that
             because no-one admires me. But I'm not
             sentimental – and, Ruth, this – self-ness, all
             the little pieces for the jigsaw – 'that doesn't
             fit who I am', 'that's not me'– that sort of
             integrity is a tiny, private quality. Out here
             – the world – it doesn't do much good. I'm
             saying why lose sight of the higher idea for
             the sake of the bits and pieces?

             Let me take off the ministerial hat. I
             want the government to pay for your new
             building. Whatever funding you've got,
             fine, but you're a way off and what if we
             make up the deficit – absorb the Elizabeth
             Institute as a public asset, bankroll its
             new premises and then use it as a shining
             example of what this country can do.

RUTH   And how long might that take to achieve?

FLINT   I'll have the confirmation in a month.
             And when we announce that we're curing
             dementia, I want to talk about you – and
             me – and I want to talk about women.
             Though given we're both white, I'm not
             sure we're necessarily going to [get the
             reaction we hope for] – though, actually, a
             woman still counts, I think – what?

RUTH   No, I – hadn't expected –

FLINT	I told you one day I'd come good. But look – did you push him? This priest?
RUTH	Push him? No –
FLINT	But you were brusque
RUTH	I was firm
FLINT	It's politics –
RUTH	It's Darwin. And politics isn't my problem
FLINT	Politics is all of our problem. So make this go away. It'd be good if you could out yourself. As a vulnerable person as well.
RUTH	And say what? Woman in a man's world?
FLINT	I meant make it about religious tolerance, you know, acceptance of each other – the doctor, she's religious too –
RUTH	She isn't
FLINT	Oh. I thought you did the candles thing on Fridays
RUTH	That was a long time ago – and my parents were alive, and my Jewishness is cultural if it's anything at all: it's not about believing anything
FLINT	Shame. Good time to talk about Jews.
RUTH	But a bad time to talk about doctors?
FLINT	It might be the right time to talk about doctors. If only you were gay. Forgive me, I don't actually know where you'd put / yourself
RUTH	I don't go in for badges, Jemima

FLINT	No, quite. It must be a tough thing to go through, this.
RUTH	Nothing compared to what the girl went through.
FLINT	No, quite. Look. You and I are going to be working together. We're on the same team once again. You deal with these problems internally and I'll step in on the external stuff. If it blows up, I mean.
RUTH	Do you think it will?
FLINT	These days, who can tell? But if it does, we can separate faith and medicine, I can say it's strange it's so often a senior woman that has abuse rained down on her –
RUTH	I wouldn't want you to risk your job, Jemima.
FLINT	I mean, I'm not declaring war on the Catholic church. Tempting as it is – but look at Martin Luther, he tried it in 1519, and here we are and he's long dead and the fucking thing's still here. Though the price of a cabinet post can't be more than
RUTH	Than me?
FLINT	Than the truth. How better to die than in a just cause.
RUTH	How best to die is – well, the whole point, really –
FLINT	If this gets bad, Ruth, I'll be there. I owe you that.

*

RUTH's house

SAMI	Why is your whole kitchen labelled? CUTLERY. BRAN FLAKES. Like did you worry that by sight alone you wouldn't know the rice was rice?
RUTH	That's funny.
SAMI	Tell your face. Am I being like more annoying than normal?
RUTH	I have absolutely no idea
SAMI	Bad day?
RUTH	Don't ever become the boss of anything. Or become really good at anything. I don't know. We evolve to fantasise about our enemies. It's evolution, the idea that the predators are coming. The rustle in the bush that might make this meal our last meal. It's a special place in our imagination. They who long to harm us. So killing them brings special kinds of joy. David screamed with delight over the corpse of Goliath. Talk to me. About something else. Your day. Anyone's day except mine.
SAMI	You'll literally never guess what I did at school today
RUTH	I'm – feeling crystal clear that you had sex.
SAMI	How do you do that? You are a witch.
	,
RUTH	where?

50

SAMI	Changing rooms. There's a weird cupboard at the back as you go through towards the swimming pool and it's like a corridor that joins together the boys' and the girls' blocks and there's a – joint toilet I think, not that it ever gets like used –
RUTH	A disabled toilet?
SAMI	Yeah
RUTH	And you and he – is it a he? – had sex in there –
SAMI	Not the first time. We did other stuff. But it's – sorry I'm embarrassed now
RUTH	It's ok, we don't have to / talk about it
SAMI	Yeah. No. I want to. It's – is it possible that I can control him? Can thoughts like move through the air like – perfume. I felt this [power] – like I had a whip wrapped round his head and it would pull and like sweep him in towards me. Like I'd cast a spell. I saw him, I had the thought and then I went there and I left the door unlocked and I sort of turned this current on in his brain – and my heart was like a – fist punching the inside of my ribcage – and I sat on the bench and – then the door was open and he's there – gripping my shoulders and he was kissing me hard like there was another person literally coming up out of him and they were like hungry like they wanted the salt off my skin and we were locking the door only it didn't lock properly so he was sort of holding it shut and then I had this

strange sense like flexing up on my tiptoes like I knew what I wanted him to do – and then he was doing it – like it was like a light I could turn on in his brain – and it was nice –

and then that was it, I was walking over the field and that was it. Next time I saw him I didn't want it. So I didn't switch it on. Time after that, this is last week, I really wanted it. So switched it on. Went to the swimming block in my last lesson and as I was walking there so was he. Like – it was like I had him on a magnet and I was just like bending him towards me. Same today. And today we –

RUTH   Had sex. Yes. [I'm a] Doctor. [and therefore] Unshockable.

SAMI   But –

but I'd brought clothes in. I knew this morning. I knew I was going to do it with him in there and I knew it was going to be at lunchtime and I knew. So I brought stuff. A dress. And other stuff. And I felt – unreal. And then I switched it on and at lunchtime

RUTH   Have you actually had a conversation with this boy?

SAMI   no.

RUTH   But presumably he won't tell / other people

SAMI   no. No way. During it he said he loved me. Felt weird that someone was saying that about me. Like it's just *me*.

RUTH	Do you love him?
SAMI	I don't know. Don't think so. How do you know? I don't know. During it he said 'I can't even look you in your eyes, I love you so much' –

*

CHARLIE	I'm sorry – I'm sorry but I can't find a knife, anywhere, sweetheart
RUTH	I know the feeling
CHARLIE	I mean it
RUTH	I know, I know –
CHARLIE	I spoke to the woman today about the thing
	I went to speak to her, today –
	I didn't mean to interrupt you.

*

SAMI	Ruth?
RUTH	Yes
SAMI	You're not saying anything. Which is like weird. Sorry. I only told you / because
RUTH	No, I'm – glad, I'm glad you told me – it's part of you
SAMI	Yeah?
RUTH	Yes

At the Institute, RUTH comes into a meeting room

RUTH	Ah. You're all here early. I wasn't aware there was a closed session.
CYPRIAN	There wasn't, Professor –
RUTH	I am, as far as I'm aware, still the Director of this Institute, and therefore Chair of the Executive Committee. Yes? / Yes. Yes. Good. Shall we open the meeting?
CYPRIAN	Yes
MURPHY	Are we really going to go through the motions like this?
RUTH	Which motion in particular?
	I propose we follow the agenda. I declare the meeting open. We are quorate, despite the usual apologies, including from Professor Creswell, who is stepping down from his post as Head of Pharmacology directly we appoint his replacement. We had sixteen applications, and our two contenders on the ballot were Doctor Bob Munro and Doctor Janet Feinman. Would anyone like to add anything further to the materials that have been circulated? No. Very good.
MURPHY	Hardiman isn't here
RUTH	No, very good, though I feel confident he will have no desire to change his vote. Would anyone here like to change their vote from the ballot you filled in

this morning? In which case. The ballot returned equal votes on both sides. Which means the deciding vote is mine and therefore that this committee has voted to appoint Doctor Feinman as head of Pharmacology. I shall propose the motion, will someone second it?

MURPHY   I'm sorry – [but]

RUTH   Apology accepted.

MURPHY   I really don't see how we can continue down that agenda when everyone in this room knows that the future of this institution is in serious question.

RUTH   Is it? Well, the next thing on the agenda is Professor Cyprian and an update from the board, / so once

CYPRIAN   Perhaps we shouldn't minute this –

JUNIOR is taking minutes

MURPHY   Why not?

COPLEY   Try listening and maybe we'll find out

CYPRIAN   The board have formally stated their – I am quoting – 'serious concerns' in a letter, signed by all of them except for three, who have sent a separate letter informing us that they have resigned.

RUTH   Resigned?

CYPRIAN   yes.

RUTH   And *this meeting* is the place to break that news?

MURPHY   I'm sorry, but this can't be a surprise –

CYPRIAN   It's *not* a surprise. I'm *furious* we've let it get
                to here. I'm disgusted that this whole witch
                hunt has been allowed to blow up – and I'm
                disgusted at the way it's being manipulated
                to achieve other ends. It's politics.

RUTH   Do people have responses to this agenda
                item?

CYPRIAN   Yes. I'd like to propose a motion, right
                now at this meeting – no, put this on the
                minutes – in support of Ruth Wolff and her
                work for this institute since its founding
                twenty years ago. And I'd like it passed
                unanimously.

        HARDIMAN comes in as MURPHY is saying

MURPHY   I'm sorry, no – I'm not going to endorse a
                statement of support because I think the
                board having resigned is a sign that we're
                getting something wrong. I think we have
                to listen. And I think we have to protect this
                Institute and work out how to persuade the
                board members to retract before / this all
                blows up –

HARDIMAN   I'm sorry to be late, everyone, but I've / got

RUTH   It's not a problem – but could we please
                keep to the agenda? Professor Cyprian
                has just told us of that some of our board
                members intend to resign –

HARDIMAN   It's not an intention. They've resigned.

RUTH   Would anyone like to respond to this item
                on the agenda?

HARDIMAN	Yes, Ruth, I'd like to ask you whether you know the reasons for the resignation, given that they're not stated on the letter –
CYPRIAN	How have you read their letter?
RUTH	I think the better question is whether there's anyone in the room who doesn't know the reasons, but we have a meeting to get on with and diseases to cure. Yes, I'm fully aware of the reasons. It's about the matter which as we all know has been the subject of some discussion,
HARDIMAN	And about which there's a petition with over twenty thousand signatures which is now well past the limit for a government response. Which is why I was late – I have / brought
CYPRIAN	I've spoken to Whitehall and they said: internal issue, nothing to do with government, [and so] they're going nowhere near it –
MURPHY	Let's see how long they can keep saying that for –
HARDIMAN	The reason I was late is / that I have
RUTH	I'm sorry, Professor Hardiman – I am sorry. This is not an anarchy, we do have an agenda and if people want to respond / to the
CYPRIAN	My response to the board's resignation is this. When Professor Wolff refused that priest access to the girl's sickbed, she was

	acting absolutely as a doctor should and we would have all behaved in the same way –
MURPHY	But you've never barred a priest from a patient
COPLEY	And neither has Ruth until this week
CYPRIAN	LOOK. This is a one-off situation. Nobody is trying to deny that people, some people, find comfort in religion, especially when we're talking about the end of life. Nobody has ever denied a priest – or a rabbi or a Muslim teacher –
HARDIMAN	An imam –
CYPRIAN	Nobody has ever denied a religious representative appropriate access to a patient when that access has been requested by the patient. But we bow to the pressure on this, when there was no clear instruction, then we're putting religion above medicine and allowing public opinion to over-ride the decision of a doctor.
MURPHY	That's not the only issue here –
HARDIMAN	The board have made it very clear to us / that
CYPRIAN	I don't want to get embroiled in repercussions and backlashes: the thing that is important here is this: to act as a doctor is to act as Ruth did. This is what it means to be a doctor. There is only one appropriate response to the board's resignation which is – again – to declare

our total and unanimous confidence in our Director – and I want that motion passed with full support.-

HARDIMAN   I'm not sure that we're clear what we're dealing with here. Ruth is a celebrity by the standards of medicine. She is visible. But we as the executive committee are here to protect this Institute. If we're going to move to this new building, we need sponsors, we need funding and support – and through that lens, this whole crisis around Ruth's conduct is a disaster.

CYPRIAN   No-one out there knows that this was Ruth –

HARDIMAN   I'm not suggesting Ruth set out to cause a problem. But this isn't about intention. The board are unhappy. The Christian community are unhappy. The girl's parents are very unhappy indeed. We cannot put out public statements in support of behaviour which has driven our Institute to the cliff-edge – and may yet push us over –

COPLEY   Forgive me, Roger, but bullshit. We ignore this and it goes away.

HARDIMAN   We *did* and it *hasn't*

CYPRIAN   So what do you propose?

HARDIMAN   The same thing I've been saying for two days – that Ruth should put out a statement of apology or go onto that programme and apologise – expressing her regret about the girl's death / and the surrounding situation –

CYPRIAN   You cannot / be serious

COPLEY   Ruth didn't kill the girl –

HARDIMAN   I didn't say she did, but public opinion is
                not on our side.

COPLEY   Vox populi over there

HARDIMAN   *(To JUNIOR.)* sorry – you, yes, I don't know
                your name, could you run and ask Rebecca
                to come up please? She's the person best-
                placed to speak to that – any objections?
                Move.

        JUNIOR goes to get ROBERTS

                but the *reason* I was *late* for this meeting, as I
                have been *trying* to say / for the last…

CYPRIAN   This is not speakers' corner. Ruth's name
                is not out there in public. We are a team.
                We are in this together. We do *not* cut
                people loose. There will not be institutional
                damage if the institute pulls together and
                that woman is the top of our field. Twenty-
                five years of sector-leading research can't
                just be *deleted* –

MURPHY   Yes it can. / It absolutely can – if she was
                subject to a malpractice suit

CYPRIAN   Over my dead body it can. Over my dead
                body.

MURPHY   Not an argument, Brian –

        ROBERTS enters

HARDIMAN   Thank you for coming, Rebecca. We hoped
                you might update us with your view of our
                current situation with the perception of
                recent events. In public.

CYPRIAN	I'm sorry, who is the chair of this meeting?
RUTH	Continue –
ROBERTS	There's articles running in two of the broadsheets tomorrow. We haven't commented – and nor has the priest. It's all anonymous so I don't think it's going to become a major story –
MURPHY	People don't like it. I don't like it – I'm sorry, Ruth – but I said that to you at the time, on the day – you got it wrong
COPLEY	Everyone knows what you think, Paul
CYPRIAN	Have the parents commented on the story?
ROBERTS	I couldn't get that info out of them
HARDIMAN	which brings me to why I was late
MURPHY	Sorry, Roger, I've been speaking to people and there is a particular sensitivity around the fact that this priest – the priest that Ruth saw fit to *push* around –
RUTH	I didn't *push* the priest
MURPHY	You absolutely did. – but part of the sensitivity, and nobody is saying it, is because he's a black man
	,
HARDIMAN	Yes –
CYPRIAN	*no* no *no no* – this is *total nonsense, I'm* a black man!
	,

61

MURPHY	Are you?
CYPRIAN	My grandmother was born in Kenya
MURPHY	it's a slightly different story when you look completely white –
RUTH	*Please*, everyone
ROBERTS	I didn't realise that – I didn't realise there was a racial element
RUTH *(chorus)* CYPRIAN *(chorus)*	There's *not* a racial element There's *not*
MURPHY	OK – but I'm the most senior person here who isn't white – who doesn't *look* white. And I don't think the way I'm addressed here is neutral.
RUTH	Neutral?
MURPHY	Neutral any more than the way you addressed the priest.

HARDIMAN very calmly addresses ROBERTS

HARDIMAN	What do you think, Rebecca?
ROBERTS	I don't know if race is [the issue] – I mean, I don't like the optics – I'm not saying it means anything but I don't like the way it looks.
HARDIMAN	I agree
RUTH	I think this might be the moment to return to the agenda – and / yes I am nonetheless aware that Professor Hardiman has been trying to address the meeting and has been continually interrupted. As heated

	as this issue has become, we owe ourselves a standard of debate. For everyone's sake. Professor Hardiman.
HARDIMAN	Professor –
	Thank you, Ruth. The reason I was late is because I have brought the father here. I've spoken to him and he's waiting in my office – I wanted him to have a / chance
COPLEY	What?
CYPRIAN	Why the hell have you got him in the building?
HARDIMAN	Because granting him the opportunity to address the executive might defuse the bomb of a screaming row in public –
RUTH	That is completely against protocol
MURPHY	Which is exactly the view someone might take of your conduct
COPLEY	Oh how many times – she didn't do ANYTHING wrong
HARDIMAN	This situation will cost us our funding and our move to our own building unless we can manage it better – and there is nobody who can speak to the girl's perspective better than her parents –
COPLEY	Everyone knows what her parents think!
CYPRIAN	Roger, you've got the father here? Not the priest?

HARDIMAN	I spoke with him myself this afternoon. He's obviously upset about the whole situation, as are we all –
COPLEY	He's asking: is it the girl's father or the holy father?
CYPRIAN	Jesus Christ –
FATHER	Amen

And they realise that the FATHER is at the doorway, played by the same actor who plays the PRIEST. It's OK if it takes the audience some time to work out which FATHER he is.

	Were you praying there? I guess that's what happens here. The name of the Lord is taken in vain because you all think you're above it. You all think you're bigger than God. Don't you?
CYPRIAN	I'm sorry if I, look, there's / not
FATHER	Keeping me sitting down there waiting for you like you're doing something important. Probably I've not got better things to do because I don't wear a white coat when I do a day's work. Fuck him. Stupid little fucking nobody with his God and his dead daughter. I could hear you screaming down the corridor.
ROBERTS	I'm going to call security
RUTH	No – it's okay – Mr Ronan / I
FATHER	You all protect each other, you people. A little fucking cabal. I've seen it on the TV, incompetence and you kill someone and then it all gets covered up. You've murdered

my little girl – and I will exact that pound of flesh – there is no way I'm going to let you write this up as some statistic – some tiny error – she was my little girl and she deserved better than this – and from all of you, counting your pennies towards your state of the art new building. You don't have a fucking clue how to treat a Catholic family –

RUTH   Mr Ronan, I'm going to stop you there. I understand that you're upset,

FATHER   Do you? Do you understand what it's like to lose your child? You got children, have you, that died?

RUTH   I wasn't saying my experience / is the same as yours

FATHER   Cut off your hand rather than go to hell. That's what Jesus said. Do you understand hell, any of you? Maggots crawling in your flesh and scalding burns and perpetual fucking torment – that is where she is. That is where she is. She died without being forgiven and she was fourteen years old and she died in mortal sin. She died. She died.

            ,

            I've got nothing to say to this lot, Roger, that I can't say to the press. I've got all the information. And I am going to scream it from the rooftops

RUTH   Mr Ronan, the decision I took as your daughter's physician / was

FATHER   It was you? You're the one who actually [did
                       it] – I thought I knew your voice. What's
                       your name?

Nobody responds

                       Someone tell me what her fucking name is,
                       would you please.

RUTH   You have no right to be in here

FATHER   Name

RUTH   My name is Ruth Wolff.

FATHER   Well, Ruth Wolff, I am going to make you
                       your own personal hell on earth. Believe
                       me. I'll dedicate myself to tearing you to
                       fucking pieces – you push people around,
                       now you get pushed around – give you a
                       taste of your own fucking medicine –

The FATHER shoves RUTH, she falls. Total chaos.

                       Fuck you all – fuck you all –

The FATHER exits

ROBERTS *(chorus)* Are you alright, Ruth?
COPLEY *(chorus)*   I'm going to call the police

RUTH   we cannot call the police. We cannot call
                       the police in the middle of this situation,
                       and I can't press charges, it'll leak –
                       (COPLEY tries to interrupt.) we cannot have a
                       police car parked *outside of this building –
                       and that is that.*

Worried looks.

CYPRIAN   I think we should adjourn this meeting –

66

RUTH	no no no No No NO. We keep *going.* SIT DOWN.

RUTH stands up.

JUNIOR	You're bleeding, Professor
ROBERTS	Ruth, you're the victim of an assault –
RUTH	I am not the victim of an anything
ROBERTS	His behaviour is something we can use, you're the victim / of
RUTH	I am not a victim and we are not sinking to that –
ROBERTS	Ruth, I can't / let you
RUTH	Sit down, Rebecca, and SHUT UP. SIT DOWN. ALL OF YOU. SIT DOWN.
	,
HARDIMAN	I didn't expect he would behave like that, I apologise for bringing him here – I thought if we listened to what / he has to say
RUTH	I need to be crystal clear. For one moment, let me be crystal clear about procedure – the chair – that is, me – that is, I am the only person here, the only one empowered to put a motion to the committee. There are two motions on the table. One proposed by Professor Cyprian, expressing absolute confidence in me, and one proposed by Professor Hardiman compelling me to make a statement of apology – and I'll put both of those forward to / the executive, but

HARDIMAN	I withdraw my motion – but allow / me to
CYPRIAN	Then put mine to the vote. Put my motion to the vote.
RUTH	Professor, please –
MURPHY	We will make ourselves look like tone-deaf imbeciles if / we don't
CYPRIAN	She founded this fucking institute
COPLEY	Calm down, Brian –
CYPRIAN	*Put the motion to the vote –*
RUTH	We've not yet formally ratified the appointment of Doctor Feinman.
HARDIMAN	When did that happen?
RUTH	Before your late / intervention, Professor.
MURPHY	Rebecca, how do you think it looks, from a PR point of view, for us to appoint *another* Jewish woman –
RUTH *(chorus)*	*another* Jewish woman?
CYPRIAN *(chorus)*	I'm sorry?
COPLEY *(chorus)*	Fucking hell
MURPHY	a *white* Jewish woman –
CYPRIAN	Can you *put* my *motion* to the *vote*
MURPHY	The reason we are having a problem with Christians is because there are hardly any of us who *work* here
RUTH	that's not why / this happened
MURPHY	and so they don't have a voice in this institute – there are people on the internet

	from the Christian community saying that *right now*
COPLEY	SHUT UP. SHUT UP. I don't want to hear the opinions of people on the internet. I really do have better things to do. But if that petition leads to an inquiry, then Ruth will be found innocent – and unlike some of you, I can say that, because I was there when the incident happened. So I say, bring it on. Let's let the procedure do its work and return the verdict we know will be returned.
MURPHY	Trigger an external inquiry ourselves, you mean? Admit it's Ruth, invite the scrutiny?
RUTH	Is that what you mean?
COPLEY	I think you're innocent Ruth, but your name's out there now. Girl's father is going to do his best, you heard him, and this is all very uncomfortable. So we have to be above board and transparent. We have to be.
RUTH	Which means handing me over, does it?
COPLEY	I – well, Ruth, I wouldn't quite put it / [like that]
RUTH	I'm sure you wouldn't
COPLEY	I'm not trying to insult you, Ruth, I'm / trying to solve
HARDIMAN	Can we return to the agenda?
	,
RUTH	Of course we may.

HARDIMAN	This isn't personal, Ruth, it really isn't personal. But the function of this committee is to protect this institute and the institute is in serious jeopardy. We are getting it wrong. I would like to propose a motion of no confidence in Ruth Wolff.
RUTH	Thank you. Before I put your motion to the executive, Professor, perhaps you might give an outline of the conversation we had in which you attempted to use this situation as a lever to persuade me to vote for Doctor Munro.
	,
HARDIMAN	This meeting becomes ever more extraordinary. I'm happy to say now – for the minutes – what I said to you in private. I offered, on the day, to take over that patient. I'm a Catholic. So was she. And this is a real issue – whether certain types of patient need certain types of doctors to attend them – but you refused without a second thought, exactly as you have refused before when this same question has been raised –
RUTH	It's called leadership
HARDIMAN	It's called management – and this has not been managed. We have a petition with – how many signatures?
ROBERTS	Over fifty thousand now
HARDIMAN *(chorus)*	Thank you.
CYPRIAN *(chorus)*	Sorry, what are you trying to imply?

70

HARDIMAN	I told Professor Wolff that this institute was seen as an exclusive Jewish organisation, which historically has been more the case than it is now – but our history and our director and many of the foundations that fund us create an impression that there are certain types of person allowed in –
COPLEY	And those types of people are Jews?
HARDIMAN	You know exactly what I mean: we are seen as an elite –
COPLEY	I cannot believe these arguments are being made with a straight face
HARDIMAN	So – how many Jews on our board?
RUTH	Now there's a question with a dark history
COPLEY	I'm sorry, I wasn't aware we were a restricted species –
CYPRIAN	Professor, could you come to your point
HARDIMAN	I told Ruth that it would be good for us to appoint a black, Catholic doctor, because it sends the message clear as day that this institute is open to all the types of people she upset –
MURPHY	exactly
COPLEY	and given that the doctor in question is the godparent to your kids –

This angers HARDIMAN and his argument really starts to burn, this now heats up

HARDIMAN	Which has absolutely nothing to do with it. She *dismissed* me out of hand.

RUTH	Because she couldn't see any integrity in your proposal
HARDIMAN	Because Ruth Wolff can't see it doesn't mean it isn't there –
RUTH	You also implied that the petition could be made to disappear if I did so. I told you then and I *stand by it now*, that I would vote for the most capable doctor and that is exactly what I have done –
HARDIMAN	The most capable doctor *in your opinion*
RUTH	I thought it might be clear it was my opinion given that it was my words in my voice emerging from my body –
HARDIMAN	I offered help and you declined. And now look where we are. We have a major crisis on our hands and this Institute is about to be embarrassingly dragged face down through the mud in full view of the medical world. Everything exposed. And *why?* Because you treated this priest with your trademark disdain, a disdain that attends to particular groups, and a disdain that is the culture of the way this building runs – not so much a *culture* as a cult: a cult of personality –
MURPHY	I second Professor Hardiman's motion of no confidence
RUTH	It hasn't been proposed yet
HARDIMAN	Then *propose* it

,

RUTH	As Professor Hardiman points out, clearly I have not done everything in my power to protect the institute from the onslaught of spiteful public attention – unwilling as I am to sacrifice my integrity on the altar of political expediency –
MURPHY	I don't think that is / a reasonable
RUTH *(sharp)*	I don't think I had finished speaking, thank you, Doctor. I could have done more to protect the reputation of this institute among those who now are crying outrage. I will therefore take the appropriate action myself and, *until* this matter can be cleared up, resign as the director of the institute

Total uproar, all the below at the same sort of time –

CYPRIAN	What?
MURPHY	It has to be put to the vote –
ROBERTS	No it fucking doesn't, if / she wants to resign she can
HARDIMAN	I don't think that – I don't know if
MURPHY	Leaving us to pick up the pieces
COPLEY	Are you sure, Ruth, is that really the way to / resolve this

CYPRIAN bangs on the table until they all go quiet

CYPRIAN	Are we to understand, Professor Wolff, that you have resigned the directorship of this institute?

,

RUTH	Yes
CYPRIAN	In which case, I believe the way it works is that the role of Director will be filled on an acting basis by the deputy director, the responsibilities of which include – in the immediate – the chairing of this meeting –

HARDIMAN stands up

HARDIMAN	Thank you, Professor.
	I believe before we move to the bigger, public questions facing us, we should discuss who will manage Professor Wolff's department and research responsibilities until such a time / as
RUTH	I will. I've resigned the directorship, nothing more.
MURPHY	The suspended director of this institute cannot continue to / work at
COPLEY	Who was suspended? She resigned
MURPHY	Not of her own volition
HARDIMAN	Can we please bring this meeting to order
RUTH	I'm going to ask for leave from my department until this case can be resolved if the Acting Director will grant me it –

Micro-beat pause

HARDIMAN	Granted.
RUTH	Then I shall commence my leave
COPLEY	I'm coming with you

ROBERTS	Me too –
RUTH	Let's not give these gentlemen everything they want –
COPLEY	I'm not giving them you, Ruth
RUTH	Thank you, Michael. Good evening, everyone.
COPLEY	No – you don't, you do not – [go through that door]

COPLEY

if we let that woman go through that door,
we open ourselves up to a poison which
could warp the nature of this profession
for years and years to come – and this
might be the turning point, this might be
where we choose. We cut her loose and let
them have her – and have her as white or
a Jew or godless or a woman – we let her
be anything other than a doctor, if we let
them drag in biography, if our identities,
if doctors' identities are put on the table,
then let's be clear what that means, because
it's Jewish doctors for Jewish patients and
fat doctors for fat patients and 'should
you perform the surgery if you haven't
undergone it yourself?', before every minor
procedure a speech from the consultant,
like teenage singers on TV talent shows,
about how 'Today's surgery is dedicated
to my poor dead grandma who really
supported my dream to be a doctor, and
would be so proud of me for operating
on today's patient' and not one bit of it
will do a thing to make us better doctors
or get better results for our patients or in

CURING THIS FUCKING DISEASE. If we do not stem the bleed of this biographical nonsense then it will drown us in a flood of blood types and birthplaces and the kind of things we like to do in bed.

If we bow to this pressure we WILL NOT GET BACK UP.

She is a DOCTOR. That is all that counts. That is the single qualification and it's handed out by teaching hospitals, not by people sitting in their back bedrooms and screaming into the internet. And if we countenance this, because of the pretended outrage of some pack of sanctimonious non-entities, we delay the work of this institute – and of this first-rate doctor – for a net gain of absolutely nothing. And the patients are the ones who will suffer.

HARDIMAN   Doctor Copley, have we reached the end of your performance? Thank you, Professor Wolff.

RUTH leaves

COPLEY   You cannot just dump people into piles. And not for nothing but there is really nobody, no human being on this earth that does not defy that sort of simplistic bullshit with their technicolour, thousand-fold complexity. And last time we chopped up the world into identity groups, let's remember where that road led – with tattoos on people's wrists –

                  and as a Jew, I get to make that point.

COPLEY leaves.

CYPRIAN	I don't think we have a quorum any longer, Professor –
HARDIMAN	*(To J.)* Let's return to the agenda – and restart the minutes, thank you. Could you close the door, please?

*

CHARLIE	What are you doing?
RUTH	I am still sitting here, in the car, trying to work out what to do –
CHARLIE	It's been three hours. How's it going?

*

JUNIOR	I need it back.
RUTH	It's got my name on it. It's got my name
JUNIOR	I need it back.
RUTH	I can't give you it back. You didn't give me it. I gave me it – I did found / the institute
JUNIOR	I know. You've resigned.
RUTH	I've resigned from the executive, not from the department –
JUNIOR	No-one thinks you're coming back
RUTH	I am coming back
JUNIOR	Right. Well, until then, I need your pass.
RUTH	I'm going to drive away now. What are you frightened of? That I'm going to break in during the night and illicitly cure people?

	Doctors having to sit around idle, chatting among the unexpectedly healthy?
JUNIOR	It isn't my decision.
RUTH	It's above your head. Of course. Hardiman? Who you working for?
JUNIOR	It's whom. For whom are you working? In case you care about language at all.

,

| RUTH | You told the patient, didn't you, that – the priest had come for her? |

,

JUNIOR	I didn't agree with you.
RUTH	Well, it wasn't your decision to make.
JUNIOR	but it should have been Emily's choice.
RUTH	God, men always think they know best – so you decided it was up to you to pick between faith and medicine?
JUNIOR	No – I chose between faith and atheism. He might have been able to comfort her. Keeping him out would not have saved her life – she was always going to die –
RUTH	And so you let her die confused and panicked, entirely without *peace*, slamming her head against her pillow – well, many congratulations, that really must feel good –
JUNIOR	If the priest had got to her earlier, perhaps that would never have happened –

RUTH	She was FOURTEEN years old –
JUNIOR	I disagree with what you did. And how you treat people. And the fact that you haven't said sorry. Can you please just hand me your pass.
	Thank you.

*

There might be an interval here – if there is, it's important that RUTH stays on stage. When the play resumes, SAMI enters. We're at RUTH's house. She has a phone.

SAMI	When I saw it I literally died
RUTH	You didn't literally die
SAMI	What?
RUTH	Literally means literally, not figuratively – in fact the whole point of the word literally is so that we can indicate that we're not speaking figuratively. It's a word to say that a *thing actually happened.* Use literally figuratively and you've successfully destroyed the whole purpose of the word. So when I say that the people I work with are literally fat fucking ignorant pigs wandering around on their hind trotters, you now don't know whether I actually work with medical pigs or whether I'm just speaking figuratively.

,

SAMI	Who did that to the car?
RUTH	What?

79

SAMI	There's a swastika. Sprayed on it.

,

RUTH	Well, it wasn't me testing out a new paint colour, if that's what you mean.
SAMI	Saw the cat out there, but it didn't look guilty. Ruth, what's going on?
RUTH	Nothing
SAMI	The phone's unplugged
RUTH	Is it?
SAMI	Who phoned you?
RUTH	If I wanted to talk about it, I'd talk about it.
SAMI	Mum –

And they both hear that word –

	I mean, I didn't – Ruth – sorry, I didn't actually realise that
RUTH	It's fine, it's fine – it was a slip of / the [tongue]
SAMI	Yeah, no, yeah it was

,

SAMI	Shall I make you some tea?
RUTH	Are you having some? / No, you don't 'do' it
SAMI	No, thank you

,

	I read the story online. Are you okay?
RUTH	I am trending.

There is something dangerous about her

which as a present participle is both ugly and inelegant.

When the end comes, it shows itself first in the language.

What are they saying?

| SAMI | You don't need to hear it |

| RUTH | The only acceptable response is that I die. This is public hanging for the digital age, hands-rubbing, a community ready with boiling tar and feathers. The crowds are assembling and I have to be purged. Joe McCarthy caught me with the reds. Goody Nurse has seen me with the devil. Fling me out beyond the city walls. Because it's only by pushing people outside your boundaries that you work out where your boundaries even are. There were death threats, Rebecca told me that. It's *over* when there's a body. Maybe that is what's required. |

| SAMI | Ruth – I don't know if you're joking or not? |

| RUTH | I'm not. The witch has to die for the story to end. |

| SAMI | You're talking about suicide – |

| RUTH | If I get there, I'll call the ambulance first, there's no danger of you being the one that finds me. No, I promise you, if I kill myself, I won't leave the clear-up to you. |

Atmosphere is getting dangerous

SAMI   I wasn't asking for that [reason]

RUTH has taken the phone

RUTH   But these people, these barely-informed
                fucking people – you want to make a
                difference do you? – you want to get a
                reaction? Do something well. Actually
                achieve something and then maybe you can
                put your real names on it

*RUTH suddenly destroys the mobile phone and it really shocks SAMI
who doesn't know how to react*

                ,

The phone is in little pieces. A calm. SAMI doesn't know what to say.

SAMI   Well, I hope you're insured

RUTH   Insurance to a doctor is like water to a fish

                ,

SAMI   Maybe – maybe we should put some music
                on.

                Okay? Okay. I'm going to just press play
                and whatever's there can play

*SAMI puts some music on. It plays for a while. RUTH laughs. And
then.*

RUTH   This isn't my music, it's Charlie's, and I'm
                afraid it is filed under the category 'music
                that makes me want to kill myself'.

The music is still playing

CHARLIE	And what is it about this track that makes you want to kill yourself?
RUTH	it's either the music or the lyrics
CHARLIE	Sarcasm. Thought of as the lowest form of wit.
RUTH	Karaoke is the lowest form of wit
CHARLIE	Don't be so bloody joyless, come on, woman –

with a bit of ad lib – CHARLIE makes RUTH dance – she's not naturally given to it, but she does give in and it's okay – in a gentle, sweet way they're happy – and the music keeps playing. CHARLIE singing along with the lyrics hits a certain point and then says

I can't remember them –

I know the words to this – I know I know the words –

CHARLIE gets quite frustrated

RUTH	It doesn't matter, sweetheart, it's a nonsense song anyway
CHARLIE	It was casting its spell – you were letting yourself go
RUTH	It's perfectly nice music –
CHARLIE	Nice music for killing yourself
RUTH	Turn it off. I can't [bear to listen to it –]

Music stops

The sound of a smashing window – the two of them suddenly alert.

SAMI	What's that?
VOICE	*(Loud.)* MURDERER

A silence. They're frightened. The sound of more glass breaking.

RUTH   *(Quietly.)* Turn it off. Sit very still. Don't
                move. The door's locked, don't worry –

SAMI nods

                The town has to mark the witch.

A bang on the door

                We'll talk quietly. We'll ask questions. You
                ask one then I ask one. Favourite colour

SAMI   Purple. Favourite animal

RUTH   – koala. Favourite word

SAMI   Pomegranate.

A bang on the door

RUTH   Your turn – come on

SAMI   Favourite person?

RUTH   I –

SAMI   Too slow. And it's still me. How many times
                have you been in love?

RUTH   Once: one time. Are you happy?

SAMI   Sometimes – are you happy?

RUTH   Sometimes. What's happened to your eye?

SAMI   It doesn't matter –

RUTH   That's not a game question

Another bang on the door. They sit still.

Tell me what happened to your eye.

,

SAMI   That boy I was telling you about. Kind of
        turned weird. I'm okay. But he like pulled
        my bag today in front of people and pulled
        all my stuff out, including, like the dress
        and stuff that I told you about, make-up
        and was throwing it and like laughing,
        being – being a total prick basically. I don't
        know why but in a second it all just *changed*.

        And then he pushed me and I fell and that
        happened to my eye – I'm okay. He went off and
        I was looking at all my books and stuff on the
        floor and I didn't want to pick the dress up really
        so I just left it there so I think it's gone now

RUTH   He is not worth a single eyelash of you. I
        think he's probably terrified by what you've
        made him feel. Because you are a gold-
        standard human being and I've seen enough
        of them to know. You will look back on him
        one day – and he will seem so far below you –

Another bang on the door

        And suddenly I'm crystal clear: you don't
        apologise for who you are. You don't hide.
        So it's time that I opened the door.

SAMI   Ruth –

RUTH   (*Loud.*) Silence me, will you? Try it. TRY it.
        Here I come –

She opens the door, the sound of outdoors

        ,

	(Loud.) And there is no-one here at all
SAMI	because you don't see it, doesn't mean it's not there –

She's relieved and breathes out

| RUTH | Though I see what you mean about the car. Do you think the swastika is a reference to my Jewish roots or is does it more generally denote my alleged fascism or acc-[use] |

She breaks off as she sees it – to SAMI, the silence is worrying –

SAMI	What?
RUTH	*(Gentle.)* Stay where you are. Stay where you are.
SAMI	what? What is it?
RUTH	It's cat

,

| | and it's dead and they've put its blood onto the front door and – a baby's dummy in its mouth and left it here on the doorstep |

There may be blood on her hands

SAMI	We should call the police
RUTH	*(As in 'no'.)* There's nothing they can do for cat, I fear.
SAMI	Are you okay?
RUTH	*(Quietly.)* I'm angry.
SAMI	What are we going to do?

*

A TV Studio.

[in the original production, ONE was the actor playing ROBERTS, TWO the actor playing HARDIMAN, THREE the actor playing MURPHY, FOUR is CYPRIAN and FIVE is JUNIOR. The actor playing FLINT stays the same. The actor playing COPLEY was the host.]

HOST   Good evening. If you've seen the news this week you'll know her name – and, likely, you'll have an opinion. We're joined tonight by Professor Ruth Wolff, Director of the Elizabeth Institute – and our panel, independently convened as experts in their fields. This is Take the Debate.

Music, the panellists enter and sit down

Thank you for joining us. Tonight: Do groups really matter? And if you're thinking 'no', I'd like to know where you've been for the last century of social history: if you know any women with the vote or gay married couples or see non-white faces on your screens. Wherever you stand on the issues, this is the fact: no human is an island. We don't drive change alone.

In the studio tonight, the individuals on our panel, representing the groups with a stake in this incident, sit side by side, despite their disagreements. Is tonight's debate religion? Abortion? Is it race? Is it – should it be – simply medical ethics? What matters here is hearing all the points of view – as we take the debate.

ONE	Professor Wolff, I'm a minister and activist on behalf of CreationVoice, which is a non-denominational Christian group who works on political policy. Good evening.
RUTH	Good evening
ONE	In the current system, it's impossible to ensure that the religious beliefs of doctors don't impact on their patients, isn't it?
RUTH	I don't think it is – a doctor with a religious objection to a certain practice would state that themselves up front and recuse themselves / from having to treat it
ONE	But you didn't do that in this instance?
RUTH	No. The key point in this / situation
ONE	Sorry – why not?
RUTH	Because I had no moral objection
ONE	But also you're not Christian?
RUTH	No, I'm not –
ONE	And so you didn't feel the last rites were important. Your religious belief – your belief about religion – had an impact on Emily Ronan.
RUTH	It's nothing to do with important or not – the fact is, there was nothing to instruct the medical team to allow the priest access. The patient's own wishes – not those of her parents – but her own wishes were simply not clear to her medical team, or, of course, we would have followed them to the letter.

ONE	But you knew that her family was Christian.
RUTH	Yes – but not whether Emily was.
ONE	Your argument was that Emily could be seriously distressed by the knowledge of her impending death. Hence your decision to deny the priest access.
RUTH	That's right –
ONE	But if she was conscious enough to realise she was dying, why not simply ask her whether she was a Catholic?
RUTH	I –
ONE	Are you an atheist?
RUTH	I'm a doctor. I don't go in for groups –
TWO	I'm a medical ethicist and a lawyer, and among other things I work on behalf of the campaign against abortion. Reports suggest that Emily Ronan died of a botched abortion procedure. Did you perform it?
RUTH	I cannot talk to you about the specifics of a patient's care –
TWO	Can we hear the recording?
HOST	We can hear part of your conversation with Father Jacob Rice, who we did invite on our programme this evening and who declined to make any response. We'll hear part of it now.

We hear, from before:

RUTH	In which case I'm going to terminate it.
FATHER	I'm now going to walk calmly into Emily's room, Doctor – I'm sorry, can you get out of my way –
RUTH	Hey –
FATHER	Get out of my way –
TWO	'In which case I'm going to terminate it'. Those are your words. Was the priest trying to stop you from carrying out an abortion procedure?
RUTH	the conversation. I meant terminate the conversation. He was recording me / and
TWO	But Emily Ronan had an abortion at your institute?
RUTH	I can't give out details of Emily's care and that / was a condition of
TWO	The details are all over the press!
RUTH	That is *not* an indication that it's right for me to discuss them –
ONE	I mean, this is ridiculous – if we asked you if you cut off her hands, you'd still say 'no comment', even if you didn't – surely confidentiality doesn't extend to things that you *didn't* do?
RUTH	OK, I didn't perform the abortion, no.
TWO	Thank you. But you *are* pro-abortion?
RUTH	Yes

FIVE	So you're pro-choice
TWO	So had Emily Ronan had a Catholic doctor, he would have known that an abortion to a Catholic is a mortal sin / and
RUTH	*He* might well have taken the same decisions I did – if *he* understood that, pro-choice or anti-choice, the choice under scrutiny *here* is whether or not to see a priest.
ONE	Emily Ronan didn't get that choice.
RUTH	No, because, as her doctor, I was acting in the patient's best interests and in this instance, the best thing I could give her was a *peaceful death.*
TWO	But that isn't what she got. You were wrong.
	,
ONE	Your institute has about five hundred staff. How do you choose your doctors?
RUTH	By their ability to perform the task in hand
ONE	So someone's religion plays no conscious part in who you employ?
RUTH	It plays no part at all. We're doctors and we hire doctors. We're trying to cure a disease. The only thing that matters is qualified. We don't pry into people's lives.
THREE	I'm a senior reader in Jewish history and a specialist in the study of Jewish culture. Are you Jewish?

RUTH	I was born to Jewish parents. I don't subscribe to a religion.
THREE	… it's not a trick question, Doctor / Wolff. Many of us have noticed the ways in which attacks on you this week employ anti-Semitic tropes. You're a hugely successful, very visible, Jewish woman – and, as you'll know, there's been support from Jewish groups for your position.
RUTH	I'm not.
	I appreciate the support – but, my identity isn't the issue. I don't go in for groups.
THREE	That confuses me when nearly 65% of the doctors you employ are women.
RUTH	Being a woman doesn't put me in a group –
THREE	But a moment ago you told us your only criteria was quality. Now you believe it's OK to discriminate to have more women?
RUTH	I think most people would agree that, for women / there is a systemic imbalance in our field and that the / opportunities
ONE	I think that's fair
THREE	this week, your Institute voted to employ a doctor in a high-ranking position, and that doctor was a Jewish woman. Her gender is important, but her Judaism isn't. Why? The Jewish people are also a minority – a minority in far smaller numbers than women –

She can't resist correcting the grammar, but almost unnoticeably

RUTH	The Jewish people is a minority, yes – look, we are trying to cure dementia. We pick the best people we can get. And some of them – are women.
THREE	Are you the beneficiary of any positive discrimination? You're born to Jewish parents, so you're Jewish. You're also a woman. Why is one characteristic worth more than another?
RUTH	We don't put our doctors in groups.

Other than the pause, this next section: fast

TWO	But – wait a minute – you do when it comes to abortion.
FIVE	I don't think we need to hear more about this [i.e. from TWO]
ONE	I think everyone deserves a chance to speak
TWO	Thank you. You said yourself, you're in favour. A Christian doctor might well be opposed.
RUTH	I'm not in favour. As a doctor, I'm neutral. I'm in favour of patient choice.
TWO	But can you be neutral about abortion if you've had one yourself?
	,
RUTH	*(Fast.)* I can't *believe* you've – OK, my private life was never part of / the deal –
ONE *(chorus)*	Wow
FIVE *(chorus)*	I don't think that's / a fair question

HOST	It's up to you, Professor, which questions / you [answer]
TWO	I asked a hypothetical / question!
RUTH	yes, I had an abortion, yes it was late-term and yes I have regrets but I would make the same call again if I were making it today – and the majority of people have open minds and *understand* that people get to make their own choices – including me – though let me be clear, it's people like you / that are the root of the problem, grubbing through the bins of my teenage years and then sitting in moral judgment –
TWO	'People like me'
	I'm here to try and put / to you people's concern
RUTH	to expose my life in the public domain? That doesn't make you a hero, it makes you a tabloid journalist – with the bloodthirsty morality of the Spanish Inquisition –
TWO	Many people think abortion is a choice made *too easily available* – and in Emily's case / one that should
RUTH	Emily did it at HOME. Went online, did her research, got hold of the drugs, and aborted her baby at *home* – now had we done it, in the hospital, she'd still be with us today – so that's all thanks to the Catholic Church – and the fascist politicians they enable – pouring Luddite hatred on a procedure which, every single

	day since it began, quite literally saves *women's lives* –
TWO	I'm not going to sit here and listen to this abortion-loving propaganda –
RUTH	Abortion loving? Say that to me again. Say that to any woman who has been through that – *horror*, but let's first acknowledge that the Catholic Church, which is *morally* opposed to abortion, has been openly corrupt since the twelfth century and is now most famous for its systemic abuse of children –
TWO	You clearly feel more strongly about abused children than murdered ones –
RUTH	No-one was MURDERED, the girl would have DIED ANYWAY.
TWO *(chorus)*	wait–
ONE *(chorus)*	Then – sorry – why not *let the priest see her?*
	,
FOUR	Professor Wolff, I'm an academic, author and activist specialising in the study of post-colonial social politics. Do you understand why people are angry?
RUTH	Clearly it's fun to ride the bandwagon.
FOUR	Speaking as a black woman, the picture of a privileged white academic using physical force to get a black man out of / a room is
RUTH	I didn't use physical force –

FOUR	I'm interested that you think you can interrupt me. But I'd like to hear the recording – can we?

We hear again

RUTH	Hey –
FATHER	Get out of my way –
RUTH	You have zero authority here. I don't know who the hell you are. You want to get uppity with me, then fine. But you're wasting your time because there is really no way I'm going to let you near that child
FATHER	Don't touch me –

FOUR	So you did use physical force?
RUTH	I touched his shoulder
FOUR	I think it sounds more violent than that –
RUTH	I think you weren't there – and so it doesn't matter what you think
FOUR	It doesn't matter what I think?
RUTH	No, no more than it matters what I think about the moon landing: I wasn't there and I don't know. You can all live in your personal realities, but nobody else has to join you there.
FIVE	Let's talk about your personal reality. I'm a researcher and the chair of a nationally recognised campaign group for the understanding of unconscious bias. Had

	the priest been white, would you have acted the same way?
RUTH	Yes. Of course.
FIVE	You went to a private school, didn't you, Professor?
RUTH	I don't see any relevance / in
FIVE	How would you describe your politics?
RUTH	I'd describe them as none of your business. And this is nothing to do with the incident I came here to clarify – in which I am defined one way: as a *doctor*.
FIVE	You're defined one way. As a doctor. You're not part of a group.
RUTH	I've only said that twenty times so far this evening, but I don't think I'm part of a group, no.
FIVE	I wish that was something I was able to say. But people force me to remember the groups I belong to when I walk down the street. Society groups us: *that's the thing it does*. You get to ignore your groups – as a white woman of a certain age, of a certain class – because you're in the elite groups.
ONE	Hang on – I don't think a *woman* is an / elite group!
THREE	Elite groups, I think, need to / be [thought about more in …]
FIVE	I'm saying that the Professor gets to see her groups only when they suit her. But what if you're not white? What if you're religious?

97

	What if you're in a group which gets less status – less freedom – less privilege –
RUTH	I have absolutely no idea what you mean
FIVE	You think 'doctor' over-rules every other type of identity. But speaking *now*, in this socio-political moment, from a contemporary perspective, I disagree –
ONE	A 'woke' perspective isn't something any of us need to / hear
FIVE	This is supposed to be a variety of viewpoints, and a 'woke' perspective / might
RUTH	Oh *god*
THREE *(chorus)*	I think if we're going to talk about elite groups, there's a bigger conversation
ONE *(chorus)*	I agree / but it
RUTH	A 'woke' perspective – a 'woke' perspective – the use of language makes one want to *weep* – *woke* means *'awakened'* – from what? *from sleep?* – it sounds like you're a member of a cult, / it's the language of spiritual conversion – when in fact, it's *one view* and if that's your view, that's your view, but it's not intrinsically *better* than any other view – other people's views are not *asleep*
FIVE	Professor – I didn't use that word
	First, I didn't use the word 'woke'. She did. Second, your definition of that word is binary: you're woke or you're not. Mine isn't, my definition of what it means to be 'woke' is much more expansive.

RUTH	Right. Well, for me, a *doctor*, language is *precise* – a diagnosis has to be specific.
FIVE	So – what? you're discounting a whole history, a whole system of ideas, because you don't like the nasty word 'woke'? Woke is an attempt – and an honest attempt – to create a consciousness of people who aren't like you.
RUTH	And *this* is not about me
FIVE	It's so *upsetting* that you won't *understand*, you think you're *above* what we're saying to you. You're a doctor, yes, but you're a human being too.
RUTH	Astonishing
FIVE	Am I wrong?
RUTH	No, you're mixing things together which aren't related – and when you mix up all your colours you only get brown –
FOUR	And brown is bad, is it?
FIVE	Exactly – that's exactly / it –
RUTH	What is your problem
FIVE	My problem is educated white people shoving black people out of the way and then behaving like they have every right to do so. My problem is thousands of years of oppression and its legacies in the world we live in now, in the language you're happy to use. My problem is that you see it as my problem.

RUTH	I'm not sure I'm responsible for my ancestors
FIVE	Then who the fuck is?
HOST	I'll have to intervene here and apologise for that language – and ask you not to swear – we're live with Professor Ruth Wolff and this is *Take the Debate.*
FOUR	Professor, do you like to be addressed as Professor?
RUTH	I don't mind – it's a word like any other
FOUR	It's a word you wear that says you get to speak – isn't it?
RUTH	I didn't get that title for Christmas, it's the result of quite a lot of *work*
FOUR	But Professor, part of the anger here is about who *owns* language, who gets the right to make things mean. Who gets to choose. The guardians of the status quo. The gatekeepers who block the doors and stop us getting through.
RUTH	Us? Who is us? I'm not a gatekeeper –
FOUR	You blocked a man from getting through a door. And that action for many people was symbolic, given that he was a priest and that he was black.
RUTH	What I can't abide is this endless dividing up of people into tribes and smaller tribes of smaller tribes. You cut humanity in half enough times, eventually it ceases to exist.

FIVE	It was people like you who cut the world in half in the first place – we are at the end of a whole history of / this
RUTH	But now we all get to choose who we are –
FIVE	But everyone has bias. And none of us can switch our bias off –
RUTH	I'm – I have a little friend, comes to my house some nights in the week to do her homework, a friend of mine, she was born a boy but now, since I've known her, at this point, for her, she's a she, as far as she's concerned, you know, she wears female clothes: it's what you're saying: she gets to choose. And that is fine by me –
FOUR	And I bet you have black friends too – and that isn't what she said –
RUTH	and this idea that I somehow hate black people / – I don't even
FOUR	I'm not accusing you of hatred, we are talking about something deeper and more complicated, it's the air we all breathe, in the language we speak –
RUTH	It really is rather low-risk, isn't it, all these battles fought on the plane of language –
FIVE	Language is step one – because some of us have to push back before we get to choose, select how we are described. You don't do groups, to you it's 'political correctness', but for people who look like me, it's the right to self-determine using language.
RUTH	Words are words –

FOUR   'Words are words'. Can we hear the
                recording again?

The recording again

   FATHER   Get out of my way –

   RUTH   You have *zero* authority here. I don't
                     know who the hell you are. You want
                     to get uppity with me, then fine. But
                     you're wasting your time because
                     there is really no way I'm going to let
                     you near that child.

FOUR   You called him 'uppity'.

RUTH   Yes. Uppity. Adjective. Above one's station.
                High-handed. Yes.

FOUR   And you're aware that that word has a
                specifically racist connotation?

RUTH   No. It's an adjective that means 'above
                one's station' and 'high-handed'.

FIVE   It's a racist word – it has a history / of racist

RUTH   Well, I didn't know that – and I certainly
                didn't intend / to be

FOUR   It's not about intention. It's the act. And it
                seems to me perfectly possible that without
                intending to, you stepped into a long
                tradition of dismissing people of colour – of
                shutting down their voice

RUTH   All because of a word

FOUR   But uppity implies another word. Uppity is
                followed by a noun. For years, for hundreds
                of years, my people were referred to using

102

	that name, which is too poisonous even to speak aloud on this programme. You know the word / I mean, I think –
RUTH	In the heat of the moment, I / made a decision
FOUR	Would you mind if I continue? As a black woman, it astonishes me that you dismiss the whole idea of labels or titles or names. But I'm talking about a particular word – a single word that is one hell of a lot more than a *word*. But if words are words, then say *that* word. On this programme. Now. Call *me* that word.
	,
RUTH	My intention with that patient / was extremely clear
FOUR	I asked you to call me that word
RUTH	No
FOUR	I thought words were words.
	,
RUTH	No
FOUR	*(Quiet.)* So you do understand that there are wider sensitivities, that there is a *history* here which carries for me a certain amount of anger and for you a certain amount of guilt. You do understand on some level that there is a context bigger than this single incident.
RUTH	Yes. Of course –

	I'm completely in favour of people getting to –

,

and the truth is I'm so tired

FOUR	Me too
RUTH	and the truth is, I don't know
	I didn't mean to – it was about the patient –
FOUR	And so can we expect an apology?
RUTH	For what?
FOUR	For anything you feel might merit an apology

,

The camera pushes in on RUTH. This could be the apology.

RUTH	As a doctor, I did nothing wrong –
HOST	I'm going to go now to Minister for Health, Jemima Flint, who's arrived with us live from Westminster tonight –
FLINT	That's right, very happy to be here –
HOST	What's your take on everything you've heard?
FLINT	Well, full disclosure: I've known Ruth since I was a very junior doctor – and she was always pretty formidable. It's important to me as a senior woman in medicine that we don't victimise a senior woman in medicine – but at the same time, your panel and people in the wider country are

taking a keen interest in this case. So it feels appropriate for us to look more closely at Ruth's conduct so that in a neutral and reasonable manner we can take a clear view of what happened on the day of Emily's deeply regrettable death – so that's what we're going to do –

HOST   A formal inquiry?

FLINT draws breath –

FLINT   Yes.

*

The broadcast is over, immediately we switch to afterwards – FLINT talking to someone else

Is it raining yet out there?

RUTH   You turned on me. You turned on me –

FLINT   And what did you expect?

RUTH   That you'd stick to your fucking word

FLINT   I cannot be seen to back someone running round tipping over every sacred cow she comes across –

RUTH   DisLOYAL. DIS. LOYAL.

HOST   Ladies, could you keep your voices down – there's still an audience

FLINT   There are things more important than you. I'll fund that new building –

RUTH   Of course you will –

FLINT   and you won't be there to see it. It's the
                  thing you never understood, Professor.
                  You have to *compromise* to get yourself some
                  power, swallow a few pills because without
                  any power you are *powerless*, ergo you can't
                  DO ANYTHING. And you getting to speak
                  your truth is only worth so much – and it's
                  not as much as hospitals or nurses. That's
                  ego, not integrity. Maybe it always was.

*FLINT has slightly lost her cool. So she makes to leave and then
turns –*

                  What d'you call a leader with no followers,
                  Ruth?

                  Just an old lady out for a stroll.

*

        A taxi

RUTH   Can we stop? Pull over – stop – I'm getting
                  out –

*It pours with rain. RUTH is soaked. Perhaps she screams at the
rain. Drums. It rains and rains and rains. As it stops raining.
RUTH puts the kettle on.*

*

        RUTH's house

RUTH   You're here late

                  And you've smashed my certificates.

SAMI   'A little friend'. OK so I heard what you
                  said. And my parents didn't know and like
                  it was obvious – and – I defended you, I –

– and so everyone gets to choose who they
are except for when it suits you to *choose
who I am* – and actually isn't that exactly
what you did to that girl – like decided
she wasn't Christian because it suited what
you thought, and now I'm your next little
project – I hope you *fucking literally DIE* –

And you don't like me using that word,
but did you ever think it's maybe not that
I'm new and like wrong but that your old
way got *old* – that it's like *CHANGE* – but
no, you're right Ruth – you are like one
hundred percent right – you are *so fucking
right* but you are also *alone* – so I hope
you're happy

and just so you know, it's not a choice, it's
not like options. It's not a set thing, this or
this, it's not something you can like crush
down into a symptom – it's me –

I didn't think that was like *us* – I thought
we were […] – and yeah I smashed your
certificates. Because who even *are* you
without them?

You're at home and you're on your own
and you *know* [everything] and you're right
and I hope that you literally literally die –

RUTH   I'm sorry, Sami – come back – I'm really
               sorry.

But SAMI is gone.

       'Literally die.'

CHARLIE speaks: DAY, and then says:

CHARLIE   I don't know what day it is.

CHARLIE looks at RUTH.

RUTH   Doorbell.

CHARLIE   How long now since you saw her?

RUTH   Days and days. I don't know

CHARLIE   Longest ever?

RUTH   Yes indeed

CHARLIE   Doorbell –

RUTH   I gave her keys, remember

                      And again

CHARLIE   Doorbell –

RUTH stands up, expecting SAMI. It isn't SAMI.

RUTH   Ah. I suppose I had better let you in.

The FATHER smiles, without meaning to. He has been at the door.

                      The irony is not lost on me.

FATHER   Thank you. I didn't stay til the end of the
                      tribunal, so I haven't / heard

RUTH   Struck off. Discrediting my profession. Ten
                      years. By which time I'm too old to practice
                      anyway. So the drawbridge is up and the
                      door slammed shut. Irony. I know.

                      ,

FATHER   I'm sorry.

RUTH	Shall we have a cup of tea in the garden? There's still some light left.
FATHER	I'd like that
RUTH	It'd be an insult to thank you for telling the truth – not least as you were under oath – but what you said was [generous]
FATHER	the only thing I could have said.
	The more I think about it, the more I think it couldn't have been any different. As a priest, I couldn't have acted differently. As a doctor, nor could you.
RUTH	I did the only thing I could have done?
FATHER	– as a doctor. Yes.
RUTH	I wish you'd seen fit to say that at the tribunal.
FATHER	You and I both are the representative of a set of ideas – of the mission of a much wider group. 'The people like me. The progress of the ideas I believe.' We can't jeopardise that for one person's benefit –
RUTH	My benefit, you mean
FATHER	Or mine. My own egotistical feeling of 'I'd done the right thing'. The ideas that this [collar] stands for are sacred. If I'd said – in public – 'she was right as a doctor to turn me away', my little truth would be a wider lie. It's a million miles from personal. I'm nothing more than a dog collar.
RUTH	And I'm a white coat.

	And there was me, thinking Jesus spoke the difficult truths and let come whatever came –
FATHER	Jesus didn't live in the digital age.
RUTH	We crucify them differently now.

,

FATHER	Though that death only amplified his life – and his ideas. His suffering only highlighted all the things he'd stood for.
RUTH	Suffering's not a symbol to the person going through it. You've seen people die. It's a solo sport. And it's not very often ethereal and calm – it's scratching and struggling and bodily fluids spraying around – and then, very suddenly, silence. For all we try and scoop up our lives into a firm story, the ending is always the same. One person's worth of flesh, going cold in a zip-up bag.
FATHER	But the ending isn't always the same. In faith, the endpoint doesn't mean the end. Death's just a bump in the road.
RUTH	We're so far apart, you and I, aren't we? Body and soul.
FATHER	Every person is a city full of people. We all contain a thousand different selves, and – they can't all be equally important. We choose which selves we want to put in charge. You've got medicine. I've got God. Something – one thing – rises to the top.

RUTH	Medicine is faith. God, I used to say that to my juniors. What's the difference between a criminal assault and a surgical procedure?
FATHER	I don't know –
RUTH	A qualification in medicine.
FATHER	Or – only one of them is an act of love.
	It's a warm night
RUTH	My hands are stone. I haven't spoken to anyone like this for a long time.
	I might smoke a cigarette. Join me, by all means. Only don't be surprised that a doctor smokes.
FATHER	Doctors smoke. God lets bad things happen. We love our parents, but we put them in homes. We love nature, but we will destroy it. 'People' isn't simple.
RUTH	I bet that's not a thing you say on Sundays.
FATHER	not everything's worth saying. Even honesty is a relative good.
RUTH	Oh, tell that to medicine. 'The patient cannot be lied to.' But does the truth fill us with hope? Hope is the silver bullet. One day someone will do a study, use numbers to prove how effective it is and – it will change everything. If a lie means hope, that lie could save your life.
FATHER	In my line of work, we've known that a long time.
RUTH	Well you should have told us

FATHER	Well you should have listened.
RUTH	Yes
FATHER	Difficult to *hear* each other over all the history, crashing around us like waves
RUTH	It's so hard, isn't it? So, so, so hard.
	I want to say I – I didn't see your colour, your race / when
FATHER	It - it isn't what you saw. It's what you didn't see. Or wouldn't see.
RUTH	And *(clicks her fingers)* I'm a racist. Final diagnosis.

The FATHER looks at RUTH. He's gentle but firm.

FATHER	The good news is: it's always been a treatable condition. A dose of humility. Some learning: learning to see the history you're standing on. Learning to be gentle when you're handling the bruises. Learning to see how much harm has been done.
	,
RUTH	I have – I mean, I will. I know: it's not just black and white

She realises, too late, closes her eyes – he smiles. And then:

FATHER	Except - the times it is.
	,
RUTH	Here's a question –
FATHER	Yes?

112

RUTH	You couldn't have read the last rites over her body.
FATHER	No. When you're dead, you're dead. You have to be alive. A hundred bishops could pour holy oil over the body and chant the sacrament in full ceremonial regalia – and your sins are still your sins. It's an apology, a forgiveness before you leave
RUTH	an apology before the end –
FATHER	or when you fear it's ending –
RUTH	Yes.

,

	I feel things are ending. The post-war institutions, the post-war ideals. The public good that blossomed after peace. All the things they fought for. Starting to crack.
FATHER	I like being here at the end of a period. Who wants the golden age?
RUTH	Does it feel like faith is ending?
FATHER	It feels like it's shedding a skin. Finding new forms. It terrifies me sometimes. But then, that's God's gift – the turning world. Forward motion. You keep going to find out the ending, trying to find the beauty in the mystery 'til you do.
RUTH	Only sometimes the mystery is boring. The days all run over and into each other – these days. I garden. People still look at me strangely in the supermarket. I try and read but it's hard.

FATHER	Hard to re-enter the real world?
RUTH	I think it's my first visit. I'm not sure I like it. How could I? I've had a human heart beat like a bird in my hand. I've held a new-born baby we'd already pronounced dead as she clicks her eyes open and cries. I've seen old eyes stretching upwards in their final minutes, breath rattling as life rolls away, one old man's skin blossoming into gooseflesh in the moment of death, halfway through the punch-line of his joke. Smile still on his face. As a doctor, you stare right into human existence. Watching it begin and end, begin and end, begin –
	and we end up in those wide, white corridors, all of us end up there, watching the ceiling spool over our head, rolled along a corridor, under the horrendous lighting – it's waiting for us, the hospital. The starting line and the end of the story. The final date on the gravestone. We should build hospitals as beautifully as churches.
FATHER	says the doctor to the priest.
RUTH	From above we're opposites, but there, we're the same. When you're old and lying on a ward, it's not mystery you'll want, but doctors. You're not the priest then. You're the patient. I'm saying, in the end, it's me you'll come to when you have your heart attack.
FATHER	And it's God you'll pray to when someone you love dies.

RUTH	I didn't, actually. Pray. I didn't pray.
	'when someone I loved died'.
	I've spent the last decades of my life fighting a brutal, ugly, merciless disease. Alzheimer's is [terrible] – well, I'd take cancer anyday. Your brain's a tall set of drawers with all your memories laid in, the most recent up here, ink still wet on the paper, down to baby's first ladybird at the bottom – and that disease sets a fire burning hot on the top. Your short-term memory's the first to go to ash, then the flames eat their way down through the drawers – and before you know it, you have really no idea who you are. No memories, no history – no you.
	Not that we made it to total oblivion. Charlie, my partner, was still lucid half the time, though not remembering – and I had to put fences up, gates, like for a toddler, all the knives in a room and lock the door sort of thing – I'd come in and the hobs would be turned on, if you can imagine that, the smell of the gas – and it was in a more lucid moment that a decision was apparently made that the way the story ended, where the line was drawn, was going to be a matter of – well – choice.
FATHER	Charlie – it was suicide?
RUTH	You probably aren't familiar with the exit hood.
FATHER	No

RUTH   Thick plastic bag goes over your head. Big
              elastic band round your neck. You take
              enough sleeping pills to knock you out.
              You hold the band tense. You wait – to fall
              asleep. It chills my blood. A hypoxic death,
              is the medical [term]. Charlie did some
              research, met with a woman who knew the
              routine, read a hundred things online. I
              had – completely inadvertently – planted
              the seed: someone had tried the same thing
              on the ward, I talked about it at home – and
              then, years later, I come home late and –

              that music is on and the kettle's cold.

              and I remember there was a plastic bag on
              the kitchen worktop and I suddenly realise
              that's it gone – and what it was for.

FATHER   You'd talked about it, the two of you?

RUTH   Can you imagine? No. The goodbye would
              have been impossible. There was a letter.
              But we knew, I think. I think we knew.

              ,

FATHER   And you were the one who found

RUTH   the body? No. I heard the music, I felt the
              kettle. I was crystal clear: I knew. I made the
              phone call – and I waited for the knock on
              the door.

              It's only when the people arrive that you
              realise your person is gone. Their little
              place now vacant. I remember walking out
              later that morning, 5am or something, I

could see them taking croissants into a hotel, all in a little basket.

And Charlie   was   dead.

That plastic bag had sat on there for days. I don't know if I looked at it and didn't recognise what it really was because I didn't want to know. I don't know if the reason I didn't know is genuinely because I didn't know.

FATHER   Charlie didn't want you there – at the end? Present, I mean –

RUTH   I wasn't invited. With my career, too many ways I could have got hold of pills, and Charlie chose a method to protect me from blame. It's manslaughter. You have to be alone: you can't be touched, you can't allow anyone in. Better not even to be in the room.

FATHER   you really think they would have come down on you / if?

RUTH   Yes.

FATHER   Because?

RUTH   Against the law. And I'm a doctor.

FATHER   you're a person too

RUTH   I think I'm a doctor more.

*

CHARLIE   You shouldn't say that

RUTH   And you shouldn't have killed yourself

CHARLIE	I couldn't have forgotten us, sweetheart. I couldn't come to that.
RUTH	I wanted to be there at the end
	I wanted to be there
	Every time a memory is accessed it is *eroded*, worn away, and so by remembering you I am forgetting you. At this point you're a virus in my brain – and I don't see the present because I'm chained to the past, the perfect past, the action complete, the thing *gone*. I'm not here.
CHARLIE	Me neither.
RUTH	And I'm not funny any more. You thought I was funny.
CHARLIE	Do you miss me or do you miss you?
RUTH	What's the difference? I miss the way you looked at me. I miss what you saw. I miss having a million dimensions.
CHARLIE	When you did what you did, what might your patient have gained?

RUTH walks to the kettle and switches it on. It starts to boil.

RUTH	A peaceful end

CHARLIE smiles as if 'see?'

CHARLIE	And
RUTH	And hope, I suppose.
	False hope.

CHARLIE   I'm not sure there's such a thing. Hope's
                 hope, isn't it? [If] you feel it then it's there

                 ,

RUTH   Oh Charlie I miss you so much

She, for the first time, sobs.

The kettle clicks off.

*She looks up and CHARLIE has gone. She looks at the plastic bag,
folded neatly on the table. She touches it.*

                 ,

*RUTH is on the phone. We shouldn't know whether this scene moves
forward in real time, or takes us back round to the beginning.*

          which

          which is it

          Hello, yes, sorry – my name is Ruth Wolff,
          double-f

          which is it (god, you'd think I'd know this)

          which is it I need if someone's died? a body,
          yes –

          no, not urgent – I'm sure. yes. Yes. I'm
          crystal clear.

          I'm a doctor

It ends